MCQ'S IN MIDWIFERY

Written by

NESTER KADZVITI MURIRA

MCQ'S In Midwifery

1st Edition

About the Author

Nester Kadzviti Murira has a PhD in Health with a focus on Adolescent Sexual and Reproductive Health from Birmingham City University, UK. She obtained a Masters' Degree in Medical Education from University of Dundee, Scotland, UK. She studied Research methodology at Sheffield University. She has a Bachelor of Education in Adult Education Degree from University of Zimbabwe and a Diploma in Nurse Education from University of Zimbabwe. She is a Registered Nurse and Midwife trained in Zimbabwe.

Nester has worked as a midwifery tutor in Zimbabwe, a Reproductive Health lecturer and a researcher with interest in Adolescent Sexual and Reproductive Health and prevention of morbidity and mortality in that age group. She is an author of several Midwifery Books, health Education Books and other contemporary topics.

With love for my grandchildren; my best buddies!

This book provides a valuable source of revision questions in Midwifery

1.Which statements are True of events in the female cycle?

a) The Follicle Stimulating Hormone produced by the anterior lobe of the pituitary gland stimulates the ovarian cycle.
b) During ovulation, there are high levels of estrogen in a female.
c) The Luteinizing hormone is produced by the ovaries.
d) Oxytocin hormone, from the posterior lobe of the pituitary lobe causes contraction of the uterus during menses.
e) The Growth hormone and Follicle Stimulating Hormone are essential hormones at puberty in females

2.Which hormones are responsible for the following body changes at puberty?

a) Growth of breasts in females?
b) Pubic hair and beard?
c) Pimples and blackheads?
d) Excessive sweat?
e) Masculine thighs and broad shoulders?

3.The female monthly cycle is controlled by hormones. Which statements are true?

a) Half way through the female monthly cycle,small amounts of the Luteinizing Hormone are produced by the anterior lobe of the pituitary gland.
b) The Luteinizing hormone causes the ripening of the growing follicle containing the ovum
c) Estrogen is produced by follicular cells in the ovary in the first half of the female monthly cycle.
d) As the follicle ripens, it produces progesterone the hormone which causes the ovum to mature.
e) Progesterone stimulates menses

4.The following are the effects of progesterone. Which statements are True?

a) Progesterone causes increase in blood supply to the pelvis and uterus.
b) Progesterone increases the production of mucus in the female genital system.
c) Progesterone changes the texture of cervical mucus from thin mucus to thick sticky mucus.
d) A woman can actually feel the flow of mucus through the vagina as a result of increase in progesterone in the female blood.
e) High levels of progesterone cause the maturation of the ovum.

5. Which statements are false?

a) At *ovulation* a girl has a smooth skin, lovely complexion and a pleasant mood and is generally attractive to the opposite sex. and displays behaviors to be noticed by the opposite sex.
b) When ovulation occurs the corpus luteum fills the empty follicle.
c) The Corpus luteum produces progesterone.
d) At the time of ovulation, the woman's body temperature rises.
e) Around ovulation, the female body is highly stimulated and the desire for sexual intercourse is increased.

6. Which statements are true of the events around the ovulation period?

a) The ovum is pushed along the fallopian tubes by peristaltic movements.
b) The ovum is pushed down the fallopian tubes by cilia.
c) The ovum is alive and active in the female internal sexual organs for at least seven days after ovulation.
d) A woman who has unprotected sexual intercourse around ovulation, is unlikely to fall pregnant
e) The cervical mucus around ovulation inhibits motility of spermatozoa.

7. Which statements are true?

a) Progesterone increases the thickness of the walls of the uterus and

the blood supply to the uterus.

b) Progesterone causes fluid accumulation in the breasts.

c) The Montgomery's tubercles appear at ovulation.

d) The nipples become prominent due to effect of progesterone on

smooth muscle.

e) The levels of estrogen are at the lowest during menses.

8. Which contraceptive method would you advise a client to try if :

a) She is over weight

b) She experiences severe headaches

c) She only has intercourse once a month when the boyfriend visits

d) She is a young and an early starter

e) She has had eleven pregnancies and has five children alive?

9. Which of the following statements are true of contraceptives?

a) Prolonged use of the combined pill may cause loss of libido
b) The condom is the only method that prevents pregnancy and sexually transmitted diseases
c) Implants cause secondary infertility
d) Implants have the lowest rate of side effects
e) The pill must be taken every day at the same time

10. Sylvia complains of heavy menses after insertion of a loop/coil. How would you manage her?

a) Tell her she will have a normal period next month
b) Advise her to change the method immediately
c) Tell her she is reacting to the copper
d) Remove the loop and tell her to come back next month with the next menstrual period
e) Reassure her and advise her to observe the next two periods

11. What advice would you give if

a) A young man thinks the couple is infertile because the woman is at fault.
b) A young man will not use the condom because he is afraid of reacting to rubber?
c) A woman who is HIV positive insists she wants a baby?
d) A woman who has lost both fallopian tubes wants a baby?
e) A woman tells you in confidence she has had a criminal abortion?

12. True or false

a) When the sperm meets and fuses with the ovum, the event is called **fertilization.**
b) The whole sperm fuses with the ovum at fertilization
c) Only the head of sperm enters the ovum during fertilization.
d) Progesterone from the corpus luteum maintains or sustains pregnancy.
e) Oestrogen from the ovary sustains pregnancy

13. Which of the following statements are true about menstruation?

a) Menstruation occurs when the levels of progesterone in the body decline.
b) The corpus luteum dries off to form scar tissue called the corpus albicans or white body.
c) The menstrual flow consists of the thick internal layer of the uterus, the ovum, mucus from the inner layer of the uterus and cervix, the unfertilized ovum.
d) The menstrual flow consists of fresh blood from the uterine artery.
e) Normal menstrual flow takes at least ten days.

14. Which of the following statements are true?

a) The female cycle repeats itself every month
b) The female cycle starts at puberty and ends at the age of sixty-five years.
c) The last normal menstrual period is essential in fertility studies.
d) Last menstrual period is required to determine a woman's age
e) Last menstrual period is required to calculate gestational age

15. Is it true or false that:

a) Pregnancy can occur through contact between a boy and a girl's genitals without penetration?
b) Semen starts flowing along the male genital system as soon as a man is aroused?
c) Sexual arousal in men can be visual and tactile?
d) Large amount of semen is predictive of high sperm count?
e) Responsible sexual behavior involves abstention, self-control, and use of a condom?

16. Which statements are true of Pre- menstruation tension?

a) The tension starts a week before menses and ends at the end of the menses.
b) It is caused by increased blood supply to the pelvis causing pelvic congestion.
c) It is caused by increased blood supply to the uterine wall.
d) The endometrial wall contraction causes premenstrual tension.
e) It is caused by vigorous and rhythmic uterine contractions.

17. During menses

a) The uterine contractions are the major cause of dysmenorrhea.
b) Uterine contraction affects all the organs in the pelvis and around the uterus such as the bowel, the bladder and pelvic muscles and ligaments.
c) Constipation is common.
d) The urge to pass urine increases
e) Headaches and chills are common.

18. What evidence-based advice would you tell them about managing period pain from the statements below?

a) Activity such as any sporting activities, sprinting, jogging, swimming, and any exercises that move the legs and pelvis such as cycling, relaxes pelvic muscles and pelvic congestion..
b) A hot shower, soaking in warm bath and heat applied to the lower abdomen i dilates blood vessels easing pain.
c) Warm drinks can soothe the pain.
d) Mild pain killers can be taken to relieve pain.
e) Bed rest is advisable to ease dysmenorrhea.

19. Women may easily get bacterial and fungal genital infections during menses. What advice can you give a group of eighth grade girls about feminine hygiene during menses?

a) Use clean and hygienic sanitary towels.
b) You can pack your genital system with anything that is absorbent.
c) Stay clean during menses and change the sanitary towel every two hours and when soaked.
d) Prevent unpleasant menstrual odors by washing or wiping the vulval area clean at each toilet use.
e) Wash hands thoroughly

20. Menarche is a significant developmental stage and a major event and landmark in the female reproductive history because:

a) Dates of menses help identify abnormalities in the pattern of menses.
b) A record of menses is useful should one decide to use contraceptives
c) A record of menses enables assessment of risk of pregnancy in the event of sexual abuse.
d) When planning a pregnancy, one needs to know when they are ovulating
e) Menses are a nuisance one must know when to expect them.

21. Which statements are true about some common menstrual problems

a) Precautious puberty is when a young child has her first menses very early in life from around eight years of age.
b) Precautious puberty is strongly associated with early development and maturity of organs.
c) Girls who have good nourishing diets tend to reach puberty faster than poorly fed children.
d) Girls who may not experience menarche until they are seventeen or older are likely to be infertile.
e) Late menarche may be caused by low levels of the Follicle Stimulating Hormone.

22. Which statements are False?

f) In late menarche hormonal assays must be done.
g) The hymen is a tough membrane that completely seals the vaginal canal to prevent infection.
h) A girl's late periods can be due to an imperforate hymen.
i) Imperforate hymen is corrected surgically.
j) Intermittent menses can be caused by insufficient flow of the Follicle Stimulating hormone.

23. A woman should see a doctor if

a) She experiences heavy and prolonged bleeding.
b) Bleeding is heavy and causes fainting or dizziness.
c) Her diet is poor in vitamins and iron
d) Her menses cease.
e) When she decides to fall pregnant

24. What is the meaning of the following terms?

a) Amenorrhoea

b) Menorrhagia

c) Metrorrhagia

d) Dysmenorrhoea

e) Mernarche

25. Which statements are true?

a) The month of mernache affects a girl's character or behavior
b) Severe dysmenorrhoea may be associated with primary infertility
c) Sexual abuse includes touching, fondling, patting, of an individual's body, contact with one's sexual organs either by touching or penetration or forcing oneself on an individual
d) Illicit sexual assault without consent is punishable by law.
e) Parent child communication allows for a good flow of information that can unravel cases of sexual abuse.

26. Some clues to child sexual abuse could be in the form of:

a) Skin changes such as rash, bruises
b) Change of gait especially limping, which could be caused by trauma and infection especially genital sores
c) Mood changes, refusal to play with others, lethargy and absent mindedness
d) Fear of certain people, fear of male voice
e) Use of sexual language or imitates sexual act in her play

27. Which statements are true of Sexual Problems in a woman?

a) Sexual response is influenced by previous experiences, memories, emotions, associations and thoughts and the phase of the female cycle.
b) The hormone oestrogen, in the early days of the female cycle causes low sexual desire (libido) and failure to reach orgasm.
c) Oestrogen, produced in the first half of the female cycle causes thickening of mucus in the female system, muscle tension,
d) Women on combined pill may experience tension headaches, poor relaxation and poor arousal.
e) Medications for hypertension, diabetes, asthma, may cause sexual dysfunction in the female.

28. Which of the following statements are true causes of poor sexual arousal in a woman?

a) Progesterone increases the desire for sexual activity.

b) Women respond well to prolonged foreplay and may reach orgasm.

c) Fear of falling pregnant may cause tension and poor arousal.
d) Feelings of inadequacy, religious inhibitions, marital discord, anger, guilt, depression, and stressful situations.
e) Localized diseases like endometriosis, cystitis, pelvic inflammatory diseases, vaginitis may cause poor arousal.

29. **When giving client education, what would you advise a woman if she**

   a) Has been diagnosed as having hypothyroidism (low levels of the hormone thyroxine)
   b) Suffers from diabetes and nervous disorders.
   c) Is on oral contraceptives especially the combined pill.
   d) She has had surgery on female organs such as salpingectomy, oophrectomy, mastectomy and hysterectomy.
   e) She tells you in confidence that she rarely experiences orgasm.

30. **You are giving client education to a woman who has settled for**

   the Combined Oral Contraceptive Pill. What would you tell her?

   a) Your blood pressure should be checked before you can start on the contraceptive Pill and every time you need a fresh supply of the Pill.
   b) This Pill is perfect for you and works well without side effects.
   c) Take the Pill every day at the same time even when you travel.
   d) Diarrhoea and vomiting is part of how the pill works.
   e) Should you forget to take the Pill, take it as soon as you can remember.

31. **What advice would you give a woman after a pregnancy, a miscarriage**

   or stillbirth?

   a) She can try for another pregnancy immediately if she so wishes.
   b) There are limited family planning methods available to prevent unwanted pregnancy soon after delivery.
   c) Progesterone only methods are best for a breast- feeding woman.
   d) Ovulation can start within 21days after delivery; you could fall pregnant this early after a pregnancy.
   e) You can't fall pregnant if you are breast-feeding exclusively.

32. **Which statements are true of the Progesterone Only Pill (POP)?**

   a) This pill contains the female hormone progesterone.
   b) Progesterone only pill suppresses ovulation.
   c) Progesterone only pill suppresses endometrial changes in the uterus making it unsuitable for implantation to occur.
   d) Progesterone only pill causes heavy menses
   e) Progesterone only Pill may be taken by breast feeding mothers as it does not suppress lactation.

33. Which of the following are side effects of Progesterone only Pill?

    a) Amenorrhoea
    b) Sexual tension
    c) Loss of appetite, indigestion and weight loss.
    d) Premenstrual headaches.
    e) High failure rate

34. Which statements are true of Contraceptive Implants?

    a) They can be implanted under the skin of the upper arm or abdomen.
    b) Implants are slowly released into one's body continuously for five years.
    c) When implants are removed the body resumes its normal female cycle immediately.
    d) Implants work contain both oestrogen and progesterone.
    e) Implants are not suitable for breast-feeding mothers.

35. Which statements are true of the Contraceptive Injection?

    a) The most common injectable contraceptive is Depo Provera.
    b) The injectable contraceptive contains oestrogen
    c) The injectable contraceptive must be repeated every 12 weeks.
    d) It works by stopping menstrual periods completely.
    e) It can be given soon after delivery or pregnancy loss

36. Which statements are true of Combined Oral Contraceptive Pill?

    a) It contains both progesterone and oestrogen.
    b) A woman on oral contraceptives has both female hormones at the same level throughout the female cycle.
    c) The COC does not have an instant effect. For the first two weeks one needs to use another method like the condom to prevent pregnancy.
    d) Most women on COC have regular menstrual cycles but some women may experience heavy menses.
    e) Some women may experience headaches and mood changes, rough dry skin and low libido.

37. You have been asked to talk about Barrier Methods of Contraception to adolescents at a youth camp. Which true statements would you emphasize on?

a) Barrier methods prevent the male seed from entering the womb.
b) The condom or sheath, or rubber tube is the only method that prevents pregnancy and sexually transmitted infections at the same time.
c) The condom is the best method for young people who wish to prevent or delay pregnancy.
d) The condom does not need a prescription or measurement of one's structures and is readily available in shops, chemists, hospitals, GP's, health centres.
e) Wrap the condom in paper before disposing of it.

38. Which of the following statements would you include when explaining condom use to a group of young men?

a) Wear the condom when you are aroused and before the sexual act.
b) Do not use oil or jel; the condom is well lubricated.
c) Hold the top of the condom as you ease out of your partner to prevent spillage of semen onto your partner's organs.
d) Wrap the condom in tissue paper and flush it in the toilet or dispose of it in the rubbish bin.
e) Use a condom once if you so wish but It can be washed or used repeatedly.

39. What is true of the Female condom?

a) Rubber is weakened and destroyed by heat; condoms must be stored away from heat and the sun.
b) The female condom like the male condom prevents both pregnancy and sexually transmitted infections.
c) The female condom must be worn before the sexual act.
d) It is easier to wear the condom if one puts one foot on the chair.
e) One should feel the condom ring around the cervix and after the sexual act, gently pull the condom out carefully without spilling the semen on one's genital organs.

40. Which statements are true of The Diaphragm or Dutch Cap?

a) This is a rubber cap which must be fitted around the cervix by health personnel for a perfect fit
b) The diaphragm prevents the male seed from entering the womb but does not prevent one from catching sexually transmitted diseases.
c) Too small a diaphragm will cause bruises around the cervix and discomfort while too large a diaphragm will allow semen to flow into the cervix.
d) One must observe very high standards of hygiene to prevent infection of the internal organs. The diaphragm must be lubricated with a spermicidal jel on both sides. And worn before the sexual act.

41. Which statements make a diaphragm different from other rubber contraceptive methods?

a) One can have repeated sexual acts once the diaphragm is in place.
b) The diaphragm must be left in place for at least four hours after the sexual act.
c) After removing the diaphragm, wash it, dry it and powder it then store it
d) away in a dust free container.
e) It requires fitting for size at the point of purchase.

41. A woman has opted to use Intrauterine Devices. What information can you provide that best describe the IUD from the statements below?

a) An intrauterine device is best fitted when one has a monthly period, or immediately after delivery.
b) An intrauterine device is a plastic shaped like the uterus.
c) The device works by preventing implantation of the fertilized ovum in the uterus.
d) Some intra-uterine contraceptive devices are coated with progesterone and continuously discharge the hormone to preventing pregnancy.
e) Some devices like the Copper T and Copper 7 are coated with copper which is spermicidal.

42. Which statements are true about The Loop (Coil)

a) The loop is a plastic coil that is placed into the uterus during the time a woman has a period.
b) The loop can stay in the uterus for as long as the woman wishes.
c) The loop discharges a hormone.
d) Intra-uterine devices have threads that are left hanging through the vagina.
e) Use of the intra-uterine devices requires very high standards of hygiene to prevent infection of the internal organs.

43. A young couple approaches you requesting information on Tubal Ligation. What can you tell the couple?

a) This is a method that can be used by a couple that feels and agree that their family is complete.
b) After tubal ligation, a woman ovulates, continues to have her monthly periods but the egg is not fertilized.
c) Tubal ligation is final, permanent and irreversible.
d) The unfertilized egg remains in the ovaries
e) The unfertilized egg is discharged during menses.

44. Which of the following cause sexually transmitted infections?

a) Treponema Pallidum
b) Streptococci
c) Chlamydia Trachomatis
d) Human Immuno Virus,
e) Pseudomonas bacteria

45.Which statements are true about Chlamydia Infection?

a)   This infection is the most common of all bacterial STIs.
b)   Chlamydial infection causes an abnormal watery and itchy genital discharge
c)   The infection does not affect the urinary system.
d)   Chlamydial infection may lead to pelvic inflammatory disease (PID)
e)   It is the only STI that causes pain during intercourse (dyspareunia).

46. The following are true complications of Chlamydia Infections

a)   The female tubes are most affected, become swollen and may collect pus inside them causing blockage of tubes.
b)   Scar tissue formation may cause tubal stricture that may cause ectopic pregnancy and infertility in women.
c)   In men Chlamydia infection causes swelling of testes (orchitis)..
d)   Chlamydia infection in men never disturbs spermatogenesis.
e)   Chlamydia infection is a cause of male infertility.

47. You are working in a gynae clinic. What would make you suspect Genital herpes in a young woman?

a)   History of a burning sensation in the groins, buttocks, and genital region.
b)   Swollen groin lymph nodes.
c)   High body temperature, chills and cough.
d)   Painful blisters or weepy sores with patches of pus in clusters on the genital organs.
e)   History of recurrent blisters and sores from time to time.

48. Which of these statements are suggestive of Herpes Simplex Virus(HSV) infection?

    a) Suppressive Antiviral therapy can be used to prevent re-occurrences of HSV.
    b) HSV is not destroyed by antiviral therapy but stays in one's body for life.
    c) Only the infected partner should seek treatment
    d) Genital herpes can be transmitted to new-born babies during childbirth.
    e) Untreated HSV infection in the new-born can result in mental retardation and death.

49. Which of the following are typical of Syphilis infection?

    a) A painless open sore with raised margins that appears on soft tissue such as the penis, the vagina, lips, gums, under the nails and around the anus.
    b) A rash that covers the whole body including the face and neck.
    c) Paralysis of limbs and mental disturbances.
    d) Large open wounds especially on the legs appear due to poor blood flow and poor nerve sensation.
    e) In young women, history of repeated abortions, stillbirth and neonatal deaths.

50. Which features are typical of syphilitic infection in a new-born?

    a) The baby may have a rash all over the body.
    b) The baby usually has abnormal features like a saddle nose causes difficulty in breathing (snuffles).
    c) Failure to feed and chokes easily
    d) The baby can have deformed internal organs
    e) The baby is small for gestation

51. Which of the following are <u>prevention measures</u> against sexually transmitted diseases?

    a) Young people must abstain from sexual activity and delay sexual relations for as long as possible.
    b) The risk of acquiring STIs increases with the number of partners over a lifetime. One should have one uninfected sexual partner.
    c) One should use a condom correctly and consistently to prevent infection.
    d) If one has been diagnosed with a sexually transmitted infection, one has the responsibility to notify all recent sex partners and urge them to get tested.
    e) While being treated for an STI one must avoid all sexual activity and abstain from alcohol.

52. Which statement is false about Genital Warts?

a) Genital warts are caused by human papillomavirus (HPV), a virus related to the virus that causes common skin warts.

b) HPV is thought to cause cancer of the cervix and other genital cancers.

c) Genital warts usually first appear as small, hard painless lumps in the vaginal area, on the penis, or around the anus but multiply quickly and develop into a fleshy, cauliflower-like appearance.

d) One of the complications of vaginal warts is that they reduce the vaginal opening causing delay in delivery of the baby resulting in fetal distress.

e) Vaginal warts may be easily removed to prevent ragged tears during delivery of the baby.

53. Which statements are False?

a) Genital warts may cause poor post-partum haemorrhage, and slow healing of bruises after delivery.

b) A baby born to a mother with genital warts can contract the virus at delivery.

c) Genital warts on the head of the penis and under the foreskin in men can make sexual activity difficult and painful and bleed during sexual activity increasing the chances of viral transmission to sexual partner.

d) HPV vaccine can be given to teenagers from 13-15 years to prevent the viral infection.

e) After removal, genital warts are likely to recur because the virus remains in one's body

54. A young man presents at the clinic which symptoms could suggest gonococcal infection?

a) Pus-like discharge from the penis.

b) Pain or difficulty on passing urine.

c) Abscesses in the groins(bubos) and around the anus

d) Oral gonococcal infection e.g. gonococcal tonsilitis

e) Anorexia

55. Which of the following are complications of gonococcal infection?

a) Gonorrhoea causes blockage of fallopian tubes in women causing **ectopic pregnancy** and infertility.

b) In men gonorrhoea causes blockage of the epididymis causing **infertility**.

c) Gonorrhoea is resistant to antibiotics.

d) The infection can be transmitted to the baby at delivery causing neonatal gonococcus sore eyes (opthalmia neonatorum)

56. How do you diagnose Trichomonas Vaginalis infection?

a) The infected female has large amounts of offensive greenish, yellowish frothy vaginal discharge.
b) The labia are swollen.
c) The vaginal walls are swollen(vaginitis) with reddish spots.
d) The vulva and inner thighs are sore.
e) The infected person has pain when passing urine (dysuria)

57. Which Sexually Transmitted Infection causes the following:

a) Swollen urethra (urethritis),
b) Cystitis.
c) Dyspareunia.
d) Prostatitis
e) Pus discharge from their urethras.

58. Which Sexually transmitted disease

a) Is caused by close contact
b) Requires regularly shave of pubic hair
c) Is caused by a fungus?
d) Causes vulval irritation and a watery offensive, milky curds, cheesy discharge from the vagina.
e) Causes milky curds can be seen under the foreskin and itchy watery offensive discharge from the penis.

59. Which sexually transmitted disease

a) Causes itchy vulval area and increases the desire to scratch all the time?
b) Causes severe discomfort when touching the vulva and when passing urine.
c) Is common in pregnancy and in women with diabetes and HIV infection?
d) Causes itchiness of the urethra and pain and soreness when passing urine in men?
e) Is common in people who practice oral and anal sex

60. Male circumcision limits sexually transmitted diseases by

a) 60%
b) 100%
c) 30%
d) 20%
e) 10%

61. Which statements are true of Male circumcision or surgical removal of the foreskin in men

a) Must be done professionally by a surgeon to prevent infection and blood loss

b) Can be dome on any man at any age

c) Circumcision does not prevent sexually transmitted diseases but makes

   the skin tough and easy to wash.

d) Prevents micro-organisms from harbouring and multiplying under the foreskin.

e) It is the best way to prevent sexually transmitted diseases in men

62. Which statements are true about Circumcision in babies

a) It can be done soon after birth
b) It can be done after-48 hours after birth
c) It should never be done in babies
d) It heals faster than in adults
e) It is a surgical procedure requiring aseptic technique

63. Pelvic Inflammatory Disease (PID) is infection and swelling of the

Female internal reproductive organs caused by bacteria and viruses.

Which statements are true of PID?

a) Pelvic inflammatory disease affects a few women.
b) The infection is usually an ascending infection from the vagina
c) PID causes inflammatory changes inside the uterus (endometritis) inflammatory changes in the uterine tubes (salpingitis) and in the ovaries (oophritis).
d) PID rarely causes (peritonitis).
e) Only one organ can be affected at a time.

64. What is true about PID infection?

a) PID Infection is passed on from one infected partner to the other through sexual contact and can also be acquired through unhygienic habits during menses.
b) Infection may spread from other internal organs like appendicitis.
c) One may feel severe lower abdomen pain, dysuria, feverish, loss of appetite
d) There is foul smelling discharge from the vagina.
e) Pelvic abscesses or a collection of pus in the pelvis is rare in PID.

21

65. Which of the following are complications of PID?

a) Pelvic Abscess
b) Salpingectomy or removal of the uterine tube is done where pus has collected in one tube.
c) Scar tissue formation may result in tubal pregnancy and loss of the tube.
d) Peritonitis
e) Septicaemia

66. What is true about HIV Infection?

a) The Human-Immuno- Deficiency Virus (HIV) is mainly spread through sexual intercourse between men and women or between men in homosexual relationships.
b) HIV can be spread through blood transfusion, needle pricks and congenital infection passed on from infected parents.
c) Any young man who catches flues, chills, coughs and sore throats every now and then and suffers from high temperature even in the dry heat of the hot seasons could be infected.
d) Thrush in the mouth of an adult and swollen lymph nodes behind the ears are signs of infection
e) The surest way for anyone to know their HIV status is to TAKE AN HIV TEST

67. Symptoms of AIDS (Acquired Immuno-Deficiency Syndrome)

a) There is always a history of previous sexually transmitted diseases like thrush of the genitals, genital warts, boils in the groins, genital sores and genital discharge of varying types.
b) Urinary tract infection characterized by dysuria is also common in HIV infection.
c) The initial stages of the presence of disease, Aids, may present like flue.
d) There is profuse sweating at night and a general feeling of ill health.
e) The symptoms may repeat themselves several times and quite frequently.

68. Which changes occur in the body due to AIDS Infection?

a) The heart is weakened, and the client feels breathless at slight effort, feet swell it becomes difficult to control hemorrhage because the clotting factors are diminished
b) The Immune System is weakened opportunistic bacterial infections occur
c) Bacterial infections like pneumonia, and tuberculosis, Pneumothorax occur repeatedly.
d) The digestive system is inflamed, the lips become swollen and the skin peels off leaving blisters and raw flesh.
e) The skin is rough and multiple abscesses occur, the hair is thin and flowy.

69. Which statements are true?

a) A woman is most fertile from the twelfth day after a period
b) A woman is most fertile seven days after ovulation.
c) The ovum is available and active in the female genital system for a week after ovulation.
d) Couples that live apart and meet occasionally, have increased chances of missing the fertile period of the female cycle.

70. Which statements are true of causes of infertility?

a) Trying for a pregnancy at the wrong time of the female cycle.
b) Poor stimulation of the ovaries by the hormones or anovulation.
c) Maternal conditions like high blood pressure and diabetes.
d) The female tubes may be blocked due to previous infection.
e) There may be structural abnormalities of the uterus and conditions that are not favourable for implantation.

71. Some of the causes of infertility in men are:

a) Inadequate amounts of testicular stimulating hormone preventing adequate production of the male hormone testosterone
b) Deformed and weak spermatozoa that fail to reach the ovum to fertilize it.
c) The vas deferens may be blocked by previous infection.
d) Infections like HIV
e) Stress

72. Which statements are true?

a) As long as a man ejaculates semen, he can be deemed to be fertile.

b) Semen is a fluid that transports the male seed.

c) Semen may not contain the male seed if the testes fail to produce the seed.

d) After prostatectomy, a man becomes infertile.

e) Testosterone is essential in spermatogenesis and maturation of spermatozoa.

73. Arrange these steps in addressing infertility in their sequence

a) Assisted fertility should be offered to the couple
b) The man's semen is examined to see the amounts and structure of the sperms.
c) Hormonal assays), are done.
d) The couple must time their sexual activity to coincide with the woman's fertile period
e) The couple must live together continuously while trying for a pregnancy.
f) Several investigations of both male and female reproductive systems are done to exclude infections, blockages and tumours of the genital organs.
g) Supplementary hormones can be given to any of the partners who may not be producing adequate amounts of hormones.
h) The couple's reproductive system is examined.

74. While counselling a couple with a problem of infertility, the man tells you he has no problem and puts the blame on the woman. Which of the following statements can help resolve the impasse?

a) Male fertility is determined by ability to produce adequate numbers of spermatozoa and not just semen.
b) Normal sperm count should be over 50 million sperms per millilitre of semen. Figures below this count may result in male sterility.
c) The male seed must have a normal size, a normal shape and must be healthy enough to swim to meet the ovum and fertilize it.
d) The amount and thickness of semen a man produces is not a sign of fertility
e) The type of food a man eats does not contribute to sperm quality.

75. Which of the following hormones are essential in production of sperms?

a) Follicle Stimulating Hormone
b) (ICSH) Interstitial Cell Stimulating Hormone
c) Testosterone.
d) Corticosteroids
e) Somatotropin?

76. TRUE or FALSE? The following are non-coital methods of reproduction where there is infertility.

a) In vitro fertilization(IVF)
b) Gamete Intrafallopian transfer(GIFT)
c) Donor Insemination(DI)
d) Surrogacy
e) Adoption

77. What causes Amenorrhoea in a woman that has had menses before?

a) Low levels of Follicle stimulating hormones in a woman who has had menses before.
b) Pregnancy
c) Extensive surgery such as hysterectomy or oophorectomy will stop menstrual periods immediately.
d) Tubal Ligation.
e) Diseases such as tuberculosis, AIDS

78. A young woman is brought into A&E collapsed. On examination she is extremely pale. Which of the following can be the cause?

a) Ruptured Ectopic pregnancy and Abortions
b) Menorrhagia
c) Placenta praevia.
d) Post-partum haemorrhage.
e) Malaria
f) Hormone Replacement Therapy

79. What specific problems can the following types of fibroids cause in a woman?

a) Sub-serous fibroids
b) Intramural fibroids
c) Pedunculated fibroids
d) Cervical fibroids
e) Multiple intra-uterine fibroids

80. Where do fibroids grow?

a) Fibroids can grow anywhere in the uterus
b) Fibroids grow on the cervix only
c) Fibroids can grow on the body of the uterus(corpus)
d) The fundus of the uterus is not affected by fibroids
e) Fibroids can be found near the uterus

81. Which of the following hormones are associated with proliferation of fibroids?

a) Estrogen
b) Progesterone
c) Prolactin
d) Human chorionic gonadotrophin
e) Somatotropin hormone.

82. Which statements are true about Fibroids?

a) Fibroids are common in women from puberty to menopause.
b) Fibroids observed after menopause are likely to have grown during the child bearing age.
c) Excessive weight gain seems to encourage the growth of fibroids.
d) Fibroids are less common in women who have used the combined oral contraceptive and those who have delivered several babies.
e) Fibroids proliferate during pregnancy

83. Which statements are true about diagnosis of fibroids?

a) Many women may not know that they have fibroids until they are examined.
b) Fibroids cause heavy monthly period bleeding because they make the uterine muscle irregular interfering with smooth contraction of the muscle.
c) Women with fibroids may have irregular monthly bleeding
d) Women with fibroids may pass clots during their monthly period or experience severe dysmenorrhea
e) Fibroids may cause incontinence

84. A middle-aged woman describes her health problem to you. Which of the following would be diagnostic of fibroids?

a) Frequency of micturition
b) Backache
c) Severe constipation
d) Hard mass on abdomen
e) Polymenorrhoea

85. Which word describes the science of the development of a person before birth?

a) Mitosis
b) Photosynthesis
c) Embryology
d) Binary Fission
e) Fertilization

86. An individual develops from fusion of:

a) The spermatozoon and the ovum.
b) Oocytes and gametocytes
c) Male and female genes
d) Oestrogen and testosterone
e) Male and female hormones

87. Spermatogenesis or production of the spermatozoa occurs in:

a) The seminiferous tubules in the testes.
b) The interstitial tissues in the testes
c) The epididymis
d) The prostate
e) Semen

88. Which of the following statements is not true of the hormone testosterone?

a) It is essential for maturation of spermatozoa
b) It is responsible for male sexual drive
c) It promotes protein metabolism
d) It is produced by the interstitial tissues of the testes
e) It is produced during sexual intercourse

89. Which of the following are causes of male infertility?

a) Low sperm count
b) Blocked seminiferous tubules
c) Failure to ejaculate
d) Poor motility of sperms
e) Impotence

90). What are the functions of semen?

a) It nourishes spermatozoa
b) It contains the male hormone
c) It transports spermatozoa
d) It enhances sexual drive
e) It prevents impotence.

91. Where is semen produced?

a) It is produced by the seminal ducts
b) It is produced by the prostate
c) It is produced in the testes
d) It is produced in the urethra
e) It is produced by the spermatic cord

92.Maturation of spermatozoon takes place in:

a) The testes
b) The epididymis
c) The scrotum
d) The seminal duct
e) The prostate

93. The ovum, develops from

a) The Graafian follicle
b) Fallopian Tubes
c) The uterus
d) Corpus luteum
e) Fimbria

94. True or False? Mature ova and sperm contain

a) 23 chromosomes each.
b) 46 chromosomes
c) As many chromosomes as possible
d) The X and Y chromosomes
e) 21 chromosomes

95. Which statements are true? Ova contain

a) One X chromosome
b) X and Y chromosomes.
c) Two X chromosomes
d) Many chromosomes
e) No chromosomes

96. True or False? A female baby is a result of a union between

a) An X bearing sperm and the ovum
b) A Y-bearing sperm and an ovum
c) The female and male chromosomes.
d) Two female chromosomes
e) Female hormones

97. Which is true? A mature ovum is released from

a) The Graafian follicle in the female ovary at ovulation.
b) The pelvic cavity
c) The fallopian tubes
d) The uterus
e) Cilia and thin mucus in the fallopian tube.

98. During a sexual act, how many spermatozoa are released in semen

a) Several million
b) Only one spermatozoon
c) A few hundreds
d) A liter
e) 10mls

99. Sperm swim in a medium of

a) Semen
b) Cervical mucus
c) Water
d) Semen and vaginal mucus
e) Sexual hormones

100. Which of these statements are true about cervical mucus at the time of ovulation?

a) Cervical mucus is, rich in sodium chloride
b) Cervical mucus is thin and in corpius.
c) Cervical mucus forms channels, *arbo vitae* through which the sperm can swim.
d) Cervical mucus is thick and in large amounts
e) Cervical mucus is thick and jelly-like

101. If release of sperms into the female genital system occurs on

the day of ovulation. True or False?

a) The Y sperm swim faster than X sperm.
b) There are increased opportunities of one having a male child.
c) There are increased opportunities of fertilization
d) There are increased opportunities of multiple pregnancy
e) All ova will be fertilized

102. True or False? During Fertilization,

a) Only one sperm penetrates the ovum.
b) Only the head of the spermatozoon containing a high concentration of DNA in its nucleus penetrates the ovum
c) The penetrating sperm produces an enzyme, hyaluronidase to penetrate the outer lining of the ovum, the zona pellucida.
d) The sperm forms a nucleus that fuses with the nucleus of the ovum to form a single cell, the zygote.
e) The zygote contains 46 chromosomes which are composed of genes from the mother or the father according to the sex of the baby.

103. True or False? Development of a new individual starts from

the time there is union between the spermatozoon and

the ovum.

a) Repeated mitotic division begins within a few hours after fertilization
b) Within three days after fertilization there is a spherical mass of cells the morula.
c) The embryo descends the fallopian tube by the third day after fertilization to implant into the uterus.
d) The cells divide into a hollow ball of cells, the blastocyst by the fourth day of fertilization
e) Implantation occurs after seven days

104. Which of the following statements are false? During implantation

a) The outer layer of cells of the blastocyst called trophoblasts burrow into the endometrium to anchor the embryo and form the placenta.
b) The inner cell mass continues to subdivide to form a figure of eight structure with two cavities separated by a group of cells, the embryonic disk.
c) The top cavity fills with shock absorbing fluid in a sac, the amnion.
d) The cells of the lower sac form the yolk sac which disappears within the second month.
e) The double layer of cells that form the embryonic disk form the new individual.

105. Which statements are True?

a) The upper layer of cells of the embryonic disk is called the ectoderm and forms the skin and nervous system
b) The inner layer of cells of the embryonic disc is the entoderm which forms epithelial tissue and internal organs.
c) The mesoderm develops between the ectoderm and entoderm and forms the muscle, bones and connective tissue
d) Through histogenesis cells form distinct body structures in a process called organogenesis.
e) The lungs and heart are formed by the ectoderm cells

106. Complete the statements below.

a) Trophoblasts differentiate into two layers. The inner layer of cells is called the------ ----.
b) The outer layer of cells of the blastocyst is the----- --.
c) The cytotrophoblasts are also called the---------- ---.
d) Between the trophoblastic layer and the cytotrophoblast is a layer of connective tissue, the------------- --- which lines the cavity of the blastocyst or the chorionic sac.
e) The trophoblasts continue to proliferate and become finger like projections termed -------------.
f) In between the chorionic villi are tiny spaces, --------------- into which maternal blood seeps.
g) The trophoblasts branch into a villous system the------- - - which becomes the placenta.
h) Within a fortnight rudimentary blood vessels and blood cells are formed in the-------------- and continues to develop and forms a capillary network within the villi.

107. Which of these statements are true?

a) The placenta consists of trophoblastic cells which divide and subdivide like branches of a tree arranged in about 200 units
b) The placental cotyledons are arranged in lobes projecting into the lacunae.
c) At least 300-600mls of blood flows though the placenta per minute.
d) Placenta succenturiate has an extra lobe situated in the membranes
e) Retained succenturiate lobe may cause dysmenorrhea.

108. In pregnancy, the fetus is surrounded by fluid, liquor amni. Which statements are true of liquor amni?

a) Liquor amni cushions the fetus and allows the fetus free movement inside the uterus
b) Liquor amni is an exudate from the amniotic membrane
c) The fetus swallows liquour which keeps the digestive system patent and thickens in late pregnancy to become meconeum.
d) liquour amni contains mineral salts, wastes, hormones and water.
e) liquor amni is plain water that bathes the fetus in utero.

109. Normal pregnancy lasts 40weeks or nine calendar months from conception to labour. Which of the statements below are true?

a) The expected date of delivery is the first day of the last normal monthly period add seven days and nine months.
b) Babies born before forty weeks are premature.
c) Babies born after forty weeks are post mature
d) Most babies arrive on the expected day of delivery.
e) Premature labour is uncommon in the late second trimester and early third trimester.

110. Which of the following statements are true of fetal life?

a) The fetus develops its own blood which does not mix with maternal blood.
b) The fetus produces its own red blood cells and white blood cells.
c) The fetus gets its nutrients and oxygen from maternal blood through the feto-placental unit.
d) The fetus shares blood with the mother at the feto-placental unit.
e) The fetal circulation has two veins carrying deoxygenated blood from the fetus and one artery carrying oxygenated blood to the fetus

111. The temporary structures in the fetal circulation are:

a) The Ductus Venosus from the umbilical vein to the inferior vena cava.
b) The Foramen ovale, a temporary opening between the two atria of the heart of the fetus
c) The ductus arteriosus from the pulmonary artery to the aorta.
d) The hypogastric arteries.
e) The liver

112. Complete the following statements on fetal circulation.

a) Blood flows from the inferior vena cava to the left side of the heart through-- ----------------.

b) ------------carry deoxygenated blood from the fetus to the placenta for oxygenation

c) ---------------closes within five minutes of birth with increase of pressure in the heart. If it fails to close the baby's color is dusky and the baby gets blue especially during feeding.

d) ------------carries oxygenated blood from the placenta to inferior vena cava from which it flows to the heart to be pumped to the rest of the fetal body.

e) The hypogastric arteries become the----------------------after birth.

113. Which structures in the fetal circulation are described below?

a) This vessel is from the pulmonary artery to the descending aorta.

b) It carries deoxygenated blood from the head and upper limbs to bypass the lungs.

c) The two vessels branch off from the internal iliac arteries to the umbilical cord and become the umbilical arteries when they the umbilical cord.

d) It allows oxygenated blood from the inferior vena cava to flow into the left side of the heart from which it is pumped to the rest of the body.

e) They become ligaments after birth.

114. Which of these statements are true about the placenta?

a) The normal placenta at term is disc shaped and weighs one sixth of the fetal weight.

b) The placenta has two surfaces, a fetal smooth surface and an irregular maternal side

c) The fetal surface of the placenta is covered by membranes, the amnion and the chorion.

d) The blood vessels can be seen entering the placenta from the fetal side of the placenta.

e) The umbilical cord enters the placenta at the center.

115. Answer True or False about the placenta

a) When the cord enters the placenta at the edge, it is called battledore insertion.

b) Umbilical vessels may run and subdivide before entering the placenta and this is called a velamentous insertion.

c) The membranes may be folded over the decidua such as in placenta circumvallata.

d) Placenta membranacea is thin and implants deep into the decidua.

e) The above placentae pause no major problem at delivery.

116. The varieties of abnormal placentae are

a) Placenta succenturiata has an extra lobe or succenturiate lobe supplied by a small artery and vein which pass through the membranes. The lobe may be separated on delivery of the placenta and may be the cause of postpartum haemorrhage and infection.

b) Placenta accreta, occurs occasionally when the trophoblasts penetrate deep into the decidua.

c) Placenta increta implants deep into the myometrium.

d) Placenta percreta occurs when trophoblasts burrow through to the serous layer of the uterus

e) In placenta increta, percreta, and accreta, the placenta can be delivered by active management of the third stage of labor.

117. The following conditions cause Placental insufficiency:

a) Fibrin deposits on the surface of the placenta destroying villi and causing

infarcts.

b) High blood pressure

c) Diabetes

d) Large tumours of the placenta.

e) High cholesterol

118. Which of the following are not functions of the placenta?

a). Respiration

b). Nutrients transfer

c) Excretory functions

b) Endocrine functions

a) Prevention of premature labor

119. Which of the following statements are true of the feto-placental unit?

a) Substances move by diffusion from high concentration to low concentration at the feto-placental unit.

b) Complex molecules are transported by phagocytic and enzymatic action

c) Gaseous exchange takes place through diffusion between maternal blood and fetal blood in the capillarics.in the intervillous space.

d) Substances that are in high concentration in maternal blood diffuse across to the fetal blood and some are assisted by enzyme action

35

e) Maternal antibodies cannot cross over to the fetus to give it passive immunity

120. The following hormones are produced by the feto-placental unit?

a) Oestrogens,
b) Human chorionic gonadotrophins,
c) Human chorionic thyrotropin,
d) Progesterone and androgens
e) Insulin.

121. True or False. The following hormonal changes are expected

in pregnancy.

a) Increased oestrogen production increases uterine muscle mass, increases blood flow to the uterus and increases the breast mass in preparation for lactation.
b) Progesterone relaxes the smooth muscles, the venous walls and prevents uterine contractions.
c) Human Chorionic Gonadotrophin stimulates continued production of oestrogen and progesterone.
d) Prolactin stimulates the maturation of the breasts alveoli and milk ducts and stimulates milk production.
e) Human placental lactogen increases the release of glucose and availability of glucose to the growing fetus.

122. Which of the following are Presumptive Signs of pregnancy?

a) Amenorrhoea in a woman who has previously menstruated normally.
b) Nausea and Vomiting otherwise commonly known as early morning sickness
c) Pica or preference or tolerance of certain foods
d) Lower abdominal pain
e) Breasts enlargement

123. True or False. Amenorrhoea in a young woman may occur because of:

a) Hormonal imbalance
b) Stress
c) Debilitating illness or local conditions of the uterus.
d) Fibroids
e) Menopause

124. True or False. Bladder Irritability otherwise known as the honeymoon syndrome is characterized by:

a) Frequency of micturition in the first trimester.
b) Dysuria
c) Incontinence
d) Backache and vaginal discharge
e) Dyspareunia

125. True or False. The typical breast changes in pregnancy are

a) The nipple increases in size.
b) The areola becomes darker
c) Montgomery's tubercles become prominent.
d) Distension of veins can be seen.
e) There is prolific flow of milk

126. True or False. The Chloasma or mask of pregnancy include:

a) Prominent Montgomery's tubercles and dark areola.
b) The linea alba which runs from the center of the pubis to the sternum and darkens to become the linea nigra.
c) Stria gravidarum, which are white stretch marks that appear on thighs and abdomen as pregnancy progresses
d) Pimples and blackheads
e) Excessive weight gain

127. True or False. The Probable signs of pregnancy are:

a) Jacquemier's sign
b) Hagar's sign.
c) Osiander's sign
d) Braxton's Hicks
e) Bundl's ring

128. True or False. In pregnancy increase of vascularity causing a bluish discoloration of the vulva and vagina otherwise known as Jacquemier's sign is observable from:

a) 8th week of gestation onwards
b) 16 weeks of pregnancy onwards
c) 28 weeks pregnancy
d) The third trimester
e) On vaginal examination during labour

129. True or False. In early pregnancy the changes in the female genital tract are:

a) The vagina becomes soft and more distensible.
b) The cervix becomes as soft as lips.
c) There is increased pulsation felt in the vaginal fornices due to increased blood floor from 8th week of pregnancy onwards
d) The uterus enlarges and becomes globular in shape
e) Cervical mucus dries off.

130. Which features are typical of early pregnancy?

a) Body temperature remains high from the time of ovulation onwards.
b) All pregnant women experience body shivers.
c) Large amounts of Human Chorionic Gonadotrophin hormone can be found in urine
d) Nausea and vomiting
e) High blood pressure

131. When can the uterine soufflé be heard?

a) At 16 weeks
b) At 12 weeks
c) At 22 weeks
d) At 24 weeks
e) After 28weeks.

132. True or False. In pregnancy, uterus increases in size by:

a) five times
b) ten times
c) twenty times
d) fifteen times
e) Twenty-five times

133. Which statements are true about Uterine Growth?

a) Longitudinal muscles run from the fundus to the lower segment
b) Oblique muscles are in abundance in the body of the uterus
c) The lower segment of the uterus is composed mostly of circular muscles
d) There are three distinct layers of the decidua
e) The cervix is less secretive

134. True or False. In early pregnancy

a) The embryo occupies the upper part of the uterus.
b) The lower part of the uterus remains empty and soft.
c) A bimanual examination easily compresses the lower part of the uterus against the firmer fundus.
d) Internal ballotment is easily done around 16th week of pregnancy onwards
e) Braxton's Hicks can be felt on palpation from 16th week.

135. True or False? The Positive signs of pregnancy are:

a) Visualization of the fetus through ultrasound scan. 3-D scan will show the features of the unborn baby.
b) Progressive enlargement of the abdomen from 12 weeks and increase in the height of fundus.
c) Fetal movements felt around 18-20 weeks of gestation
d) Fetal Heart Sounds can be picked by Doppler around 10weeks and on auscultation after twenty weeks of gestation.
e) Palpation of defined fetal parts around 12weeks

136. The following statements are true of abortion

a) Abortion is expulsion of a fetus from the uterus before it is viable
b) Any woman can have an abortion
c) Abortion is common in primiparous women.
d) Abortion is one of the causes of maternal loss
e) Abortion may result in anemia

137. True or False. The causes of abortion are:

a) The pregnancy itself (ovofetal causes).
b) Something originating from the mother (maternal causes)
c) Causes related to the father (paternal) causes.
d) Extraneous causes
e) Excessive alcohol intake

138. True or False? Abortions that occur between 6-10 weeks of gestation could largely be due to the following:

a) Chromosomal abnormality
b) Defective implantation
c) Inadequate amounts of Human Chorionic Gonadotrophic hormone.
d) Local disorders of the genital tract such as bicornuate uterus, myomata and uterine retroversion.
e) Maternal obesity.

139. True or False. Abortion can be caused by:

a) Trauma to the abdomen.
b) Deliberate interference.
c) Stress
d) Some off the counter medications taken in early pregnancy
e) Exposure to smoking.

140. Which of the following statements are true of abortion?

a) Defects in the male chromosomes results in abortion.
b) Infectious diseases such as HIV may cause abortion.
c) Maternal pyrexia may cause abortion
d) Diarrhea and vomiting may cause abortion
e) Once one has had an abortion they are likely to have another one.

141. Which of these varieties of abortion are likely to be reversed?

a) Threatened Abortion
b) Inevitable abortion
c) Missed abortion
d) Incomplete abortion
e) Carneous mole

142. Which statements are true about a woman bleeding vaginally in the first trimester of pregnancy?

a) The bleeding may be implantation bleeding which occurs as the trophoblasts sink into the uterine wall.
b) The woman may be having a monthly period
c) The woman could be having a threatened abortion
d) The woman could have a placenta praevia
e) The woman could have a hydatidiform mole

143. Which statements are False about threatened abortion?

a) The bleeding comes from a closed cervix
b) There are no contractions.
c) Digital vaginal examination should be done.
d) A speculum examination confirms if the source of bleeding is inside the uterus.
e) An ultra sound scan establishes that the client is pregnant.

144. Which of the following statements are true?

a) When uterine contractions are strong, and the cervix is open, abortion is inevitable.
b) Abortion is incomplete when only part of the products of conception are expelled.
c) Abortion is incomplete when there are strong contractions and heavy bleeding
d) Abortion is complete when all the products of conception are expelled.
e) Spontaneous abortion has no known cause

145. List actions that must be taken when managing a woman with heavy vaginal bleeding after an abortion chronologically

    a) Give ergometrine
    b) The woman must have uterine curettage.
    c) Transfuse client
    d) Check haemoglobin
    e) Replace fluid lost
    f) Give anti-tetanus toxoid
    g) Give antibiotics
    h) Obtain thorough history

146. Induced abortion which is not therapeutic may also be referred to as Criminal or backyard abortion. What is true about criminal abortion?

    a) Objects may be used to induce abortion
    b) Induced abortions tend to be incomplete
    c) The dangers of induced abortion are haemorrhage and infection
    d) Curettage is the treatment for induced abortion.
    e) Broad spectrum antibiotics are given as a rule after induced abortion

147. A woman who has missed a few monthly periods comes into A&E. What may lead you to suspect septic abortion?

    a) Profuse active bleeding
    b) Backache
    c) Offensive vaginal discharge
    d) Hyper Pyrexia
    e) Nausea and vomiting

148. Which statements are true about septic abortion?

    a) The abortion is incomplete
    b) The abortion could be criminal
    c) The woman may have Pyrexia and offensive vaginal discharge.
    d) The uterus is well contracted
    e) The fetus may still be viable

149. True or False. The dangers of septic abortion are:

a) Infection may involve myometrium and may spread to tubes and pelvic peritoneum
b) Infection caused by E.Coli is likely to cause Urinary tract infection
c) The woman is in danger of endotoxic shock
d) The uterus is boggy and tender and fails to contract
e) There is no danger of dehydration

150. The likely complications of septic abortion are:

a) Pelvic inflammatory Disease
b) HIV infection
c) Blocked fallopian tubes leading to ectopic pregnancy and infertility
d) Renal failure
e) Endorcarditis

151. Arrange the following statements in the order you would take the actions in managing a young woman with septic abortion

a) Take high vaginal swab
b) Treat with intravenous antibiotics
c) Prepare the woman for evacuation and curettage immediately
d) Check haemoglobin
e) Rehydrate the woman with intravenous fluids to replace lost fluids

152.Answer True or False. You can suspect a missed abortion if

a) A woman has missed a monthly period
b) A woman who has missed a monthly period no longer feels pregnant
c) There is no uterine growth in a woman who has missed several monthly periods
d) There is heavy bleeding in a woman who has missed a monthly period
e) A woman who has missed a period has a dark vaginal discharge

153. Which of the statements below are true of missed abortion?

a) The embryo dies and is retained in the uterus
b) There is a carneous mole
c) The embryo disintegrates and is discharged
d) The embryo becomes a fetus papyraceus
e) The embryo can be saved

154. Which statements are False about Habitual Abortion?

a) Abortion occurs three times in succession
b) One intentionally interferes with a pregnancy three times
c) Abortion is spontaneous
d) Membranes are retained
e) Refer to obstetrician for further management of subsequent pregnancies.

155. The causes of habitual abortion are likely to be:

a) Uterine abnormality
b) Cervical incompetence
c) Interference
d) Rh incompatibility
e) Fetal abnormality

156. Management of habitual abortion may include

a) Hysterogram to exclude uterine abnormality
b) Cervical suture with subsequent pregnancy
c) Bed rest throughout pregnancy
d) Discussion on safe sexual positions in pregnancy
e) Tubal ligation

157. True or False. Therapeutic abortion can be done in the following situations:

a) If the pregnancy puts the mother at risk e.g. cardiovascular disease, malignancy, HIV Infection
b) In severe fetal abnormality
c) In the case of contraceptive failure.
d) When a woman has been raped and does not want to keep the pregnancy
e) In disputed paternity
f) In unwanted unplanned pregnancy

158. After an abortion which midwifery actions are appropriate?

a) The woman's haemoglobin levels must be checked
b) The woman must be advised on diet rich in iron and folic acid
c) Every woman must be on iron supplements
d) Discuss suitable family planning methods with client.
e) Advise on adoption

159. Which statements are False about ectopic pregnancy?

a) The fertilised ovum fails to descend down the fallopian tube to the uterus.
b) Fertilization occurs outside the uterus
c) Ovulation occurs too often
d) Implantation occurs anywhere but, in the uterus
e) There is obstruction in the fallopian tubes

160. True or False. In ectopic gestation

a) The fate of the pregnancy depends on the site of the implantation, the thickness of the area and the trophoblastic activity.
b) The fallopian tube distends and the trophoblastic action further weakens the tubal wall until it bursts.
c) Bleeding may be concealed causing a pelvic haematoma in the pouch of Douglas.
d) Bleeding is heavy where the trophoblasts erode a large blood vessel
e) Where haemorrhage is slight the pregnancy may be saved.

161. Which statements are false about ectopic gestation?

a) Fertilization and implantation may take place in the abdominal cavity in

less than 1% of women in the fimbriated end of the fallopian tube, 17%,

b) in the ampulla over 50%,in the isthmus of the tube about

c) 25% and in the interstitial portion of the uterus.
d) Implantation occurs in the lower segment of the uterus.
e) Pelvic infection by Chlamydia, gonococcus is the only cause of ectopic gestation.

162. The following are signs and symptoms of ectopic pregnancy

a) A history of amenorrhoea for 5-10 weeks
b) Sharp abdominal pain on one side of the lower abdomen.
c) A palpable mass in the lower abdomen
d) Diarrhoea and vomiting
e) The woman may have vaginal bleeding, feel pain at the tip of the shoulder, and may vomit

163.A woman is admitted into a gynae ward with a diagnosis of ruptured ectopic pregnancy. Which of the following activities would be life-saving in the management of the woman?

a) Provision of emotional support
b) Contact with the client's spouse
c) Pain relief
d) Intravenous infusion
e) Administration of oxygen

164.The following are signs of shock. True or False?

a) A very low blood pressure and a very rapid pulse,
b) Restlessness
c) Cold and clammy skin
d) Sighing respirations
e) Dehydration

165. In Ectopic pregnancy which are the life- saving actions?

a) Give Iv infusion of plasma expanding fluid to replace lost fluid and prevent circulatory collapse.
b) An emergency laparotomy to remove the pregnancy and control haemorrhage must be done.
c) Prophylactic antibiotics and a sedative must be given.
d) Discuss family planning with client
e) Offer your condolences

166. True or False? After an ectopic pregnancy

a) A woman can have successful subsequent pregnancies if the remaining tube is healthy.
b) Family planning methods must be discussed with the client.
c) Haemoglobin check must be done.
d) The client must abstain from sexual intercourse until the doctor tells her to resume.
e) A diet rich in iron is advised.

167. Which of the following <u>are not</u> objectives of Antenatal Care:

a) To identify diseases that may affect expectant women's health and the health of the pregnancy.
b) To prevent maternal and fetal morbidity and mortality.
c) To inform clients about healthy behaviours that promote good health for a successful pregnancy.
d) To provide family planning education
e) Provide relevant information to clients essential in informed decisions about the health of the mother and unborn baby

168. In the care of an expectant mother, which of the following attitudes and behaviours must the midwife adopt?

a) Empower clients with as much health information as possible according to gestation
b) Enable women to express their fears and anxiety.
c) Respond to women's health information needs with informed, useful evidence based information.
d) Explore the needs of the client and provide client-centred health information using appropriate communication Models
e) Plan, teach women what she thinks is important for women to know.

169. Comprehensive collection of relevant client history includes:

a) Demographic history
b) Previous medical history
c) Current medical history
d) Obstetric history
e) Curriculum vitae

170. Which of the following statements are true of good history taking?

a) Clearly recorded demographic history enables correct identification of clients.
b) Knowledge of area of residence is essential in assessment of health problems endemic in certain areas, and special needs in specific communities.
c) Knowledge of next of kin enables identification of clients with special needs such as single women, divorced women, destitute clients
d) Knowledge of the client's age assists in identification of teenage pregnancies, elderly primiparous women and helps health personnel to plan for relevant care for clients
e) Knowledge of parity of clients is just a formality

171. In reproductive history taking

a) Medical history reveals underlying medical conditions that may have a negative impact on current pregnancy such as epilepsy, heart disease, hypertension, diabetes, renal disease, asthma.
b) Surgical history is essential for screening for emergency surgical delivery.
c) Family history of clients is necessary in identification of diseases that run in families that may have an impact on the client and her unborn baby.
d) Present History is key and essential in management of the present pregnancy
e) Reproductive history is essential to determine if client is high risk or low risk

172. In antenatal care thorough history taking is essential in planning midwifery care and identifying risk. Which statements are true of a woman's antenatal history?

a) Medical history identifies recent acute illness, current and recent medication, and chronic illness.

b) Surgical history identifies problems with anaesthesia, genital tract surgery and other major surgery.

c) Obstetric history informs the midwife about the client's previous pregnancies, abortions, types of deliveries
e) Sexual history reveals the number of sexual partners, previous and current sexually transmitted diseases, sexual abuse, preconception contraception.

173. Which statements are true of the fundal height?

a) Measurement of the fundal height is done from the symphis pubis to the top of the fundus

b) The uterine size is used to estimate the size of the fetus.

c) Around 12weeks the fundal height should be just above the symphysis pubis.

d) The fundal height generally matches the gestation in weeks from 21 weeks to 36 weeks.

174. Blood specimens must be collected from all pregnant women for the following:

a) Haemoglobin estimation
b) Group and Xmatch
c) Urinalysis
d) HIV Test
e) Zika virus

175. A healthy pregnant woman should have the following antenatal investigations results

a) Haemoglobin<11.5mg/dl

b) Haematocrit <33%

c) Platelets 150-400,000mm

d) Negative RPR

e) Rubella Titer 1:8Immune

176. Which statements are true about the physiological changes in pregnancy?

a) The heart rate, stroke volume and cardiac output increase

b) The blood volume increases

c) Blood pressure rises and systemic vascular resistance increases

d)Glomerular filtration and urinary output increase

e) There is no change in respiratory rate.

177. In pregnancy which of the following statements are true of changes in the circulatory system?

a) The blood volume increases in pregnancy because of the changes in the myometrium and endometrium, the development of the placenta.
b) The plasma volume increases gradually from the tenth week of gestation to 50% above the non-pregnant volume by the third trimester.
c) The red cell volume increases by 30% to meet the oxygen demand in pregnancy.
d) The red cell volume increase is less than the plasma volume causing a fall in the concentration of red cells in the blood and a reduction in the haemoglobin from 13.9g per 100mls in non-pregnant woman to just over 12g per 100mls from 20weeks gestation till term.
e) .Anaemia should be considered to be present if the haemoglobin is 11gm/100mls

178. In pregnancy

a) There is an increase in white cells and platelets.
b) Cardiac output increases by 30-50% in pregnancy. The heart rate increases by about 15%
c) There is reduced peripheral resistance due to the effect of progesterone on smooth muscle.
d) There is a general venous pressure rise in the veins of the legs resulting in varicosity.

179. The causes of Anaemia in pregnancy are:

a) Inadequate iron in the diet

b) Excessive loss of iron due to infections like HIV, infestations such as

   hookworm, malaria, bilharzias

c) Heavy pre-pregnant menses, trauma, antepartum haemorrhage.

d) Malabsorption syndromes

180. Effects of anaemia on the mother are:

a) Heart disease and severe debilitation
b) Respiratory problems
c) Infections
d) Poor maternal effort in second stage of labour
e) Post partum haemorrhage

181.An anaemic woman may:

a) Have failure to breast feed successfully
b) Poor healing of wounds and recovery from illness
c) Circulatory failure (dyspnoea, tarchycardia)
d) Increase incidences of maternal mortality

182.Effects of maternal anaemia on the fetus and infant. Which statements are true?

a) Increased incidence of abortion
b) Increased incidence of prematurity
c) Low birth weight
d) Infant is prone to infections
e) Infant becomes anaemic.

183. Choose FALSE statements from below. How is Anaemia in pregnancy managed?

a) Routine haemoglobin test on registering for care
b) Repeat haemoglobin tests at 28,32 and 36weeks of gestation
c) Depending on level of anaemia and gestation, oral iron can be given where haemoglobin is around 10G
d) Encourage a diet high in iron and vitamins
e) Parenteral iron is given only in late pregnancy for haemoglobin below 10g/mmle

184. Various changes occur in the cardio vascular system because of pregnancy. Which of the following are true?

a) There is reduction of peripheral resistance and increase of blood.

b). There is an increase in pulse rate and cardiac stoke volume that increases

the workload of the heart.

c)The blood pressure lowers

d)Physiological anaemia occurs because of plasma increase by 50%

e) Increase in plasma volume causes a rise in blood pressure

185. Which grade of Heart disease in pregnancy is described below?

a) Slight exertion causes dyspnoea and comfort fatigue but client comfortable at rest

b) The client has no symptoms although signs of cardiac damage are present

c) The client is comfortable at rest but is easily exhausted on slight effort. May become breathless and have palpitations

d) The client has signs of heart disease even at rest.

e) Client is asymptomatic with no signs of disease

186. Management of heart disease in pregnancy includes the following:

a) Refer all cases of dyspnoea, slight oedema, tarchycardia to cardiologist.
b) Control of salt and fluid intake
c) Control of weight gain
d) Monitoring oedema, heart rate and respiratory rate.
e) Monitoring cardiac enzymes, electrolyte balance every week.

187. Which statements are true about body weight in pregnancy

a) Initial weight on booking for care in pregnancy provides a baseline from which to monitor and provide relevant evidence- based advice, counselling and health promotion
b) Normal pregnancy weight gain increases gradually with gestation as the fetus gains weight and liquor amni increases in amount.
c) Excessive weight gain is suggestive of conditions causing fluid retention such as diabetes, hypertension, cardiac disease, renal disease.
d) Weight loss is suggestive of famine, nutritional diseases and debilitating diseases such as tuberculosis and HIV infection
e) Maternal weight is not indicative of the fetal weight.

188. Which statements are false about significance of the height of the client in pregnancy?

a) A tall client is likely to have a problem free pregnancy.
b) A tall woman almost always has a spacious pelvis and an easy labour
c) Short clients tend to have larger babies for their pelves.
d) Short clients are associated with cephalo-pelvic disproportion and operative delivery.
e) Short clients are at high risk of malpresentation, obstructed labour and other complications requiring operative delivery.

189 .Urine testing in pregnancy is done to diagnose

a) Worm infestation in tropical environments, (bilharziasis, tape worm, hookworm) which are major causes of anaemia in pregnancy
b) Fresh blood in urine could indicate bladder or urethral infection or trauma
c) Smoky urine appearance may be suggestive of blood in urine(upper urinary tract infection).
d) Concentrated foul smelling urine is suggestive of Renal diseases
e) Sweet smelling clear urine is suggestive of glucose in urine diagnostic of Diabetes in pregnancy.

190.What is the purpose of An ultrasound scan in pregnancy care? Which statements are true?

a) Detects fetal cardiac output
b) Determines fetal position
c) Detects placental position and assesses placental function
d) Measures amniotic fluid volume
e) Measures fetal growth

191. One of the dangers that are associated with USS is supine hypotension. Which of the following are true signs and symptoms of supine hypotension?

a) Pallor
b) Nausea
c) Diaphoresis
d) Tarchycardia
e) Severe thirst

192. What measure can a midwife/sonographer take to prevent supine hypotension? Which statements are false?

a) Place a rolled towel/small rolled blanket under the right hip to lift the gravid uterus off the inferior vena cava.
b) Talk to the client all the time to find out how she feels
c) Give a glass of water before procedure.
d) Quickly perform the procedure before the client complains
e) Sit the patient in an upright position.

193. What are the true indications for amniocentesis?

a) Chromosomal analysis
b) Measure Amniotic Fluid Pressure
c) To determine fetal lung maturity by measuring Lecethin Syphingomyelin surfactant
d) To check for meconium in suspected fetal distress or postmaturity
e) To measure bilirubin level in fetal haemolytic disease due to Rh incompatibility.

194. What could be the cause of vaginal haemorrhage a woman reports around 32 weeks of gestation?

a) Abortion
b) Placenta praevia
c) Abruptio Placentae
d) Preterm labour
e) Menstruation

195. What signs might a woman report that are suggestive of Pregnancy Induced Hypertension?

a) Altered blurred vision and flashes of light
b) Nagging headache
c) Severe epigastric pain
d) Oedema of feet, face and fingers
e) Increased appetite

196. Complete the following statements. At the antenatal clinic if a woman complains of

a) Abdominal cramping, it is suggestive of------------------------.
b) Decreased fetal movements is suggestive of--------------------.
c) Persistent vomiting is suggestive of----------------------.
d) Dysuria is suggestive of---------------------.
e) Leaking fluid vaginally is suggestive of---------------.

197. Exercise in pregnancy is recommended. The midwife must advise a woman to stop exercise if:

a) She experiences vaginal bleeding.
b) She has reduced fetal movements
c) She has chest pain, dyspnoea and dizziness.
d) She is leaking amniotic fluid
e) She is not sleeping well.

198. The following diagnostic tests are done in pregnancy except for one. Which test is not essential in pregnancy?

a) Glucose Tolerence Test for detection of gestational diabetes
b) High vaginal swab for detection of group B Streptococcus
c) Fetal Fibronectin predictive of premature labor.
d) Antibody screening
e) INR

199. On abdominal Inspection the midwife must look for:

a) Skin texture(firm, tight in primipara)(Loose and flabby in multipara)rough, dry, broken, rash) and advise accordingly
b) Stretch- marks, and marked linea nigra and allay anxieties
c) Scars indicative of previous surgery and trauma and investigate the cause of scars and type of operation. Exclude physical abuse
d) Size of the abdomen is suggestive of gestation of pregnancy, IUGR, large for gestation suggestive of multiple pregnancy, hydatidiform mole, polyhydramnios.
e) Shape of abdomen is suggestive of parity(ovoid in primipara, globula in multipara).

200. The possible causes of large for dates height of fundus could be

a) Multiple pregnancy
b) Hydatidiform mole
c) Polyhydramnios
d) Obesity
e) Large meal before examination.

201. A broad Shape of abdomen in pregnancy could be caused by

a) Multiple gestation
b) Loose abdominal muscles of grand-multiparity,
c) Big baby
d) Hydatidiform mole
e) Polyhydramnios.

202. Which of these statements below are True or false about fetal movements?

a) The first fetal movements are around sixteen weeks in multiparous women and around 22weeks in primiparous women
b) Excessive fetal movements spread all over the abdomen are suggestive of multiple limbs in multiple pregnancy.
c) The absence of fetal movements at all is suggestive of hydatidiform mole, pseudocyaesis, intra-uterine death.
d) Fetal movements are stronger during the second trimester
e) Excessive fetal movements in labour mark the beginning of the second stage of labour.

203. Which statements are true about abdominal palpation?

a) Fundal palpation ascertains the part of the fetus occupying the fundus of the uterus
b) Lateral palpation is diagnostic of the fetal part that lies on the sides of the uterus, and which side the fetal back lies.
c) Pelvic palpation ascertains the part of the fetus that occupies the lower part of the abdomen.
d) Pawlik's grip is a gentle grip made using the thumb and index finger to feel for the presenting part just above the symphysis pubis
e) Walking movements using tips of fingers are diagnostic of the parts of the fetal body that lye across the abdomen.

204. The Lie of the fetus is the relationship of the long axis of the fetus to the long axis of the uterus. Which statements are true about the lie of the fetus?

a) The fetus adopts a longitudinal lie in all primiparous women.
b) Abnormalities like transverse and oblique lie occur in primiparous women.
c) The causes of abnormal lie are short cord, tumors of the uterus, shape of the pelvis, multiple pregnancy,fetal abnormality.
d) The lie of the fetus can always be corrected manually.
e) Abnormal lie of the fetus is likely to cause obstructed labor.

205. The relationship of the fetal trunk to limbs and head is called the attitude. Which statements are false about the fetal attitude?

a) The normal attitude is that of flexion. The back is bent forward, the head is flexed with the chin on the chest. The thighs are flexed on the abdomen and the legs are cross legged on the thighs.
b) In primiparous women the fetal attitude is always that of flexion.
c) The attitude of the fetus is affected by the shape of the maternal pelvis, fetal abnormalities, intra-uterine death, intrauterine tumors.
d) If the fetus adopts a military attitude, it presents with the brow.
e) In face presentation, the attitude of the fetus is that of extention..

206. Fill in the blank spaces

a) The part of the fetus that lies over the pelvic brim or the lower pole of the

   uterus is the ----------------.

b) Four presentations that may cause obstructed labour are-------------------

c) The part of the presentation that determines the position adopted by the

   fetus is the---------------------.

f) The-------------------is the relationship of the denominator to six areas of the pelvis.
g) The------------- is the part that lies over the cervical os in labour

207. Which statements are true about the fetal heart on auscultation?

a) The fetal heart is clearer where the back has been identified on palpation.
b) The fetal heart is usually around the maternal umbilical area.
c) The maternal pulse is faster than the fetal heart- beat.
d) The normal fetal heart beat is 120-140 beats per minute.
e) Fetal bradycardia means the fetus is asleep.

208. Which are the true signs of a previous pregnancy in a woman?

a) Flabby breasts and prominent nipples
b) Lax abdominal muscles and loose skin
c) Stria gravidarum and linea nigra are more marked.
d) The vulva gapes and the labia minora project infront of the labia majora and vagina is roomy
e) The cervix is closed tight and can only allow a tip of finger towards the end of pregnancy

209. Which statements are true about the objectives of antenatal client education?

a) Provide evidence based health information relevant to client's condition and health problems
a) Create risk awareness of dangerous cultural and old house wives practices
b) Explain simple and complex investigations and procedures the woman is likely to be exposed to in her child bearing experience
c) Discuss self-care based on examination findings
d) Discuss topics of interest to the midwife.

210. Which statement is false about antenatal education?

a) Informing women and their spouses about events of labor
b) Imparting baby care skills to women and their spouses
c) Discussing sexuality, sexually transmitted diseases and sexual relationships
d) Demonstrating parenting skills to clients
e) Family planning course for clients

211. Which statements are true about a hydatidiform mole?

a) This is a mass of vesicles filling up the uterus as a result of cystic proliferation of chorionic epithelium.
b) The mole can become malignant.
c) The embryo can be absorbed.
d) The mole can cause bright red or brownish vaginal discharge from around 12weeks of gestation.
e) The fetal heart beat can be heard

212. Which of the features below are false of a woman with a hydatidiform mole?

a) A woman with a hydatidiform mole may have pain and tenderness of the abdomen.
b) A woman with hydatidiform mole feels excessive fetal movements.
c) No fetal parts are detected on palpation
d) The woman may have excessive hyperemisis gravidarum
e) The client may have high blood pressure

213. A hydatidiform mole may cause serious complications to a woman. Which of the listed are complications of a hydatidiform mole?

a) Profuse Haemorrhage
b) Endotoxic shock
c) Erosion of the uterine wall
d) Choriocarcinoma
e) Endometriosis

214. Polyhydramnios is when the amount of amniotic fluid in the amniotic sac exceeds 1500mls. Polyhydramnios may be associated with:

a) Monozygotic twins
b) Fetal monstrosities such as anencephaly
c) Imperforate oesophagus
d) Diabetes in pregnancy
e) Breech presentation

215. Which of the listed statements are true of acute polyhydramnios?

a) Occurs in second trimester
b) Causes sudden acute distension of abdomen, severe abdominal pain, vomiting and tense abdomen which is difficult to palpate.
c) Spontaneous abortion may occur.
d) The woman may have pyrexia
e) The client must have emergency caesarean section

216. A Large globular abdomen on inspection is suggestive of:

a) Polyhydramnios
b) Multiple pregnancy
c) Hydatidiform mole
d) Heart disease in pregnancy
e) Obesity

217. Which statements are true about Hyperemesis Gravidarum?

a) Usually occurs in the first trimester
b) Results in weight loss, dehydration and electrolyte imbalance
c) It can be controlled by anti-emetics
d) Occurs in primiparous women
e) Is associated with fetal abnormalities

218. Polyhydramnios may cause the following symptoms :

a) Dyspnoea especially at night
b) Abdominal discomfort
c) Indigestion
d) Heartburn and constipation
e) Abortion and Premature labour

219. During labour, polyhydramnios is likely to cause:

a) Cord Prolapse
b) Malpresentations
c) Postpartum haemorrhage
d) Strong uterine contractions
e) Early engagement of presenting part

220. The following conditions put women at risk in early pregnancy

a) Haemorrhage
b) Intra-uterine growth retardation
c) Severe infections
d) Hyperemisis gravidarum
e) Frequency of micturiction

221. In mid pregnancy a woman is at risk if she has

a) Urinary Tract infection
b) Hypertension
c) Marked chloasma
d) Anaemia
e) Heart disease

222. During labour a woman is at risk if

a) Her blood pressure is high
b) She has uterine inertia
c) she vomits
d) She bleeds heavily
e) She has tarchycardia

223. The fetus is at risk if

a) The heart rate ranges between 120-140 contractions
b) There is meconeum stained liquor
c) There is compound presentation
d) The head remains high despite good contractions
e) The cord prolapses

224. The following are obstetric emergencies

a) Bundl's ring
b) Haemorrhage
c) Eclampsia
d) Uterine inertia
e) Cord presentation

225. Premature labor is onset of labor before 36 weeks .Answer True or False about the causes of premature labor.

a) Any condition that causes maternal high temperature such as malaria, urinary tract infection
b) Sexually transmitted infections such as syphilis, HIV/ AIDS
c) Hypertension and eclampsia
d) Abnormal uterine structure and uterine growths
e) Incompetent cervix

226. Answer True or False. Premature labour can occur because of

a) Fetal abnormalities
b) Placenta praevia
c) Polyhydramnios
d) Multiple pregnancies
e) Hormonal insufficiency

227.The midwife must consider the following measures in the management of premature labour. Answer True or False

a) Refer to hospital for immediate care by obstetrician
b) Exclude infections like malaria, HIV
c) Perform a vaginal examination before referring patient to hospital
d) A gentle speculum examination is done to assess cervical dilatation
e) Observe and record contractions

228. Which statements are True about Cord Prolapse?

a) Cord prolapse occurs in spontaneous rapture of membranes especially where the presenting part is high and not engaged and where the presenting part is irregular and does not apply well to the cervix like the buttocks in breech presentation
b) The prolapsed cord may be compressed by presenting part causing suffocation of the fetus.
c) Cord may fall out into the vaginal vault or it may dangle out between mother's leg where it may go into spasms once exposed to different temperatures
d) The cord may pull on the placenta causing early separation of the placenta, antepartum hemorrhage, and suffocation of the unborn baby
e) With continuous flow of liquor, the unborn baby is exposed to ascending infection.

229. In managing cord prolapse, arrange the actions a midwife must take in appropriate order

a) Prepare and refer for surgery without delay.

b) Do not pack the vagina with pads this increases chances of infection and may cause spasms of the cord.

c) Position expectant client appropriately, left lateral position with pillow in between legs and one pillow under the hip. Cover client's legs from hip to prevent lowering temperature.

d) Inform client about the situation without causing undue anxiety

e) Monitor fetal heart every 10-15 minutes

230. The following are true signs of obstructed labour

a) Poor application of presenting part to cervix

b) High head with strong contractions

c) Shoulder presentation

d) Deep transverse arrest

e) Maternal distress

231. The following are signs of fetal distress

a) Early deceleration of fetal heart with abnormal baseline

b) Excessive fetal movements

c) Meconeum stained liquor

d) Poor decent of presenting part

e) Brardycardia

232. Abruptio Placentae is premature separation of the placenta which may be complete or incomplete. Which clinical findings are true of abruptio placentae?

a) Sudden onset of localised abdominal pain

b) Firm board like fundus

c) Vaginal bleeding

d) Alteration in fetal heart rate

e) Strong contractions

233. Which actions should a midwife take in management of abruptio placentae?

a) Monitoring signs of shock
b) Evaluating fetal heart rate
c) Do vaginal examination to ascertain source of haemorrhage
d) Initiate IV therapy
e) Prepare for Caesarean section.

234. Placenta Praevia is a low- lying placenta which may dip into the lower segment partially or completely cover the internal os. Which of the following are the clinical features of placenta praevia?

a) Painless vaginal bleeding
b) Post coital bleeding
c) Soft abdomen on palpation
d) No alteration to fetal heart rate
e) Strong contractions

235. In cephalo-pelvic disprortion, which of the following statements are false?

a) The presenting part engages in the pelvic brim in late pregnancy
b) The presenting part may not engage
c) There is poor decent of presenting part
d) The fault can be with both the passages and the passenger
e) The fault is with the powers

236. Ultrasound scan is a radiological diagnostic investigation. Which statements are true of the purposes of ultra-sound scan in early pregnancy?

a) To exclude ectopic pregnancy where there is discomfort in the abdomen in early pregnancy
b) To diagnose or confirm a pregnancy (Diagnostic Scan) within the first 8 weeks after missing a normal monthly period
c) To confirm when the baby is due especially where one is not sure of when they fell pregnant (Dating Scan)
d) To obtain information about the sex of the baby to enable parents to decide on names, decide on colours of clothing to buy in advance or just to know what baby they are expecting.
e) To identify fetal abnormalities especially where there is excessive vomiting (hyperemisis gravidarum).

237. In mid and late pregnancy why would an Ultrasound scan be done?

a) To locate the position of the placenta in the event of bleeding in pregnancy (antepartum haemorrhage)
b) To confirm multiple pregnancy and identify the number of babies in a pregnancy.
c) To see the baby's real features and not just a dark image using 3D scans especially in the last trimester
d) To inform health personnel about the size of the baby and the position adopted by the baby in late pregnancy.
e) To detect some obvious fetal abnormalities.

238. What is the purpose of an ultrasound scan in labour?

a) To make decisions on how the baby can be delivered.
b) To diagnose causes of prolonged first stage of labour
c) To exclude obstructed labour
d) To diagnose tumors of the pelvis
e) To confirm the sex of the baby

239. In the Second Trimester, the fundal height can assist in the diagnosis of fetal growth. What would an increase in fundal height may be suggestive of?

a) Normal fetal growth
b) Multiple pregnancy,
c) Polyhydramnious
d) Macrosomia
e) fetal abnormality

240. Why may there be insignificant fundal height growth in a pregnant woman?

a) IUGR
b) Fetal abnormality
c) Maternal malnutrition
d) Fetal death
e) Pseudocyaesis

241. Which of these are common medical complications in the second trimester?

a) Hyperemisis gravidarum
b) High Blood Pressure
c) Anaemia
d) Diabetes
e) Placenta praevia

242. Which statements are true of pre-eclampsia?

a) Pre-eclamptic syndrome is characterised by high blood pressure, oedema and proteineuria
b) Pre-eclampsia is common in primiparous women
c) Pre-eclampsia may cause placental insufficiency
d) Pre-eclampsia may lead to eclampsia
e) Pre-eclampsia is associated with prematurity

243. What are the true signs of imminent eclampsia?

a) Persistent headache
b) Dizziness and seizure activity
c) Blurred or altered vision
d) Epigastric pain, nausea and vomiting
e) High blood pressure

244. What laboratory signs are typical of the HELLP Syndrome of Eclampsia?

a) Haemolysis
b) Elevated Liver Enzymes
c) Low Platlets
d) Proteinuria
e) Low Blood sugar.

245. Which are the Four causes of haemorrhage in pregnancy?

a) Placenta praevia
b) Abruption placentae
c) Trauma to the genital tract
d) Abortion
e) Menses

246. Placenta praevia is associated with:

a) Chance implantation
b) Large placenta especially in uniovular twin pregnancy
c) Uterine Fibroids in the fundus
d) rand-multiparity
e) Fibrinogenaemia in the mother

247. Which are the true facts about placenta praevia from those listed below?

a) The bleeding is accompanied by severe backache and lower abdominal pain
b) Bleeding is bright red with clots
c) Bleeding is spontaneous and painless
d) The blood may trickle out or can be retained in the abdomen
e) The bleeding is from the mother

248.What grades of placenta praevia are described below?

a) The tip of the placenta is in the lower segment of the uterus
b) Half the placenta lies in the lower segment
c) The placenta extends to the internal os
d) The placenta lies over the internal os

249. Which among the listed are the causes of abruptio placentae?

a) Trauma like a blow to the abdomen
b) High blood pressure
c) Short cord
d) Cord round the neck or limb
e) Big baby

250. Which statements are true of abruptio placentae?

a) Bleeding is always internal and retained in the abdomen
b) The abdomen is hard and board like
c) The abdomen is soft and easy to palpate
d) There is always history of trauma to the abdomen
e) There are signs of internal haemorrhage

251. Identify true statements about management of antepartum haemorrhage from the five below.

a) The fetus is in danger therefore fetal monitoring must be done strictly.
b) Bleeding is from both the mother and the fetus the midwife must monitor closely.
c) The midwife must always raise the foot of the bed
d) A vaginal examination must be done four- hourly
e) Delivery must be done immediately

252. What are the immediate dangers of antepartum haemorrhage?

a) Fetal and maternal loss
b) Shehaan's syndrome
c) Anaemia
d) IUGR
e) Pain

254. One of the causes of maternal debilitation is anaemia. What are the clinical signs of anaemia?

a) Palor of mucus membranes of the mouth and tongue

c) Severe weakness and breathlessness

c) Dysuria

d) Tarchycardia

e) Low blood pressure

255.The midwife's role in management of clients with anaemia in pregnancy includes:

a) Offering advice on diet rich in iron and calcium supplements in the first and second trimester.
b) Referring clients with anaemia in the third trimester for further management
c) Checking clients' haemoglobin monthly
d) Excluding infections such as malaria, bilharzias, HIV and other debilitating conditions
e) Refer anaemic clients for appropriate management

256. A midwife should suspect and investigate for gestational diabetes in the following situations

a) When an expectant client has excessive weight gain
b) When a client has undue and abnormal fundal height increase
c) When a client complains of polyphagia, polyuria, polydipsia, fatigue, itchy vulva
d) The client has history of previous large babies
e) The client goes into premature labour

257.The causes of cord prolapse are:

a) Polyhydramnious

b) Early rupture of membranes

c) Malpresentations

d) Exercises in pregnancy

e) Multiple pregnancy

258. The role of the midwife in antenatal education in the second trimester is to:

a) Discuss habits and practices in second trimester of pregnancy. Discourage habits detrimental to health of mother and baby like high alcohol consumption and smoking.
b) Discuss beliefs and cultural practices in second trimester
c) Discuss Sex in late pregnancy and comfortable sexual positions
d) Ensure that client has relevant information and understands investigative procedures

259. The following are obstetric emergencies. True or False?

a) Gestational diabetes, hypertension, anaemia, heart disease.
b) Antepartum haemorrhage,
c) PIH,
d) Eclampsia, abruption placentae,
e) Cord prolapse.

260 The midwife has an obligation to familiarize her clients in the third trimester with:

a) Massage and breathing techniques in labour
b) Positions used in labour and child birth
c) The onset of labour, signs of labour, the stages of labour, procedures done in labour, analgesia in labour
d) Hyperemisis gravidarum
e) Family planning methods

261. Which statements are true about managing a Cardiac patient in labour?

a) Nurse in an upright position
b) Analgesics should be given. Avoid barbiturates
c) Oxygen should be given if breathless
d) The client should have assisted delivery with forceps
e) The third stage of labour must be actively managed.

262. The management of the Puerperium in the cardiac patient is as follows:

a) Grade 3 and 4 must be closely monitored.
b) The client must be nursed in upright position
c) Oxygen must be handy
d) Prevent infection that may cause further complications like bacterial endocarditis
e) Grade 3 and 4 must have tubal ligation.

263. In Potential Diabetes what are the true facts from the list below?

a) The client has a family history of diabetes.
b) The client has delivered a child weighing 4kg or more
c) The client has delivered an unexplained stillborn child.
d) The client has lost weight
e) The client has glucose in urine

264 Which of the statements below are true of Gestational Diabetes?

a) The body instead burns fat to produce energy. The fat oxidation is incomplete producing ketoacidosis.
b) In pregnancy there is a delay in the transfer of glucose from blood to tissues. High levels of glucose are found in blood.
c) Blood glucose levels are increased by the presence of oestrogen and progesterone as well as human placental lactogen which oppose functions of insulin.
d) Insulin resistance decreases as pregnancy progresses. Glucose however is not readily transferred to the fetus.
e) Diabetes is found in about 2% of unsuspected pregnant women and may disappear between pregnancies.

265. Which is true? A woman with Latent Diabetes

a) Has a normal Glucose Tolerance Test
b) Has had an abnormal blood glucose test before
c) The client is obese
d) This client is likely to develop Diabetes long after a pregnancy
e) The client likes sweets and cakes

266. A woman with Chemical Diabetes(subclinical or asymptomatic)

a) Has an abnormal Glucose Tolerance Test (GTT)
b) The client has no symptoms of diabetes
c) The client is obese
d) The client has a family history of diabetes
e) The client has pruritis vulvae

267. A client with Clinical Diabetes

a) Has symptoms of diabetes
b) The client's GTT is abnormal
c) The client craves sweet food
d) Has glucose in urine
e) May have monilial infections

268.What are the effects of Diabetes on Pregnancy? Answer True or False

a) Monilial infections are common
b) The client has an increased rate of Pre-eclampsia increasing fetal mortality
c) The client may have Polyhydramnios
d) The fetus is likely to be small for gestation
e) Congenital malformations are increased

269. What are the effects of pregnancy on Diabetes? Answer True or False.

a) Pregnancy increases the severity of diabetes.
b) Intra-uterine deaths due to ketosis increase
c) Fungal infections increase
d) Control of diabetes becomes difficult
e) Pregnancy reduces the client's rate of metabolism

270. The following statements are true about the management of a client with diabetes. Answer True or False.

a) Maintain low blood glucose towards pregnancy term.
b) The client must be under the care of a physician,an obstetrician and a paediatrician.
c) The client can eat anything she likes in large amounts to cater for the growing fetus
d) The client must be seen at antenatal clinics more often and must expect hospitalization anytime during pregnancy.
e) Close fetal heart rate monitoring should be done and complications are looming, delivery should be effected from 32 weeks gestation

271. Answer True or False. If a woman's gestational diabetes is well controlled

a) Trial of normal labour may be attempted
b) There should be close monitoring of the fetal condition
c) Prolonged labour must be avoided
d) The client must have a glucose bolus every now and then
e) Caesarean section must be done where there are signs of fetal and maternal distress, rising Blood pressure, hypo and hyperglycaemia.

272. Answer True or False. Post- delivery care of a woman with gestational diabetes should include

a) Continuous monitoring of the client's blood glucose levels
b) Fungal and bacterial infections must be treated
c) The client must be advised on managing her diet
d) The client must be assisted to manage her medication.
e) Urinalysis and blood glucose monitoring may not be necessary post delivery

273. Answer True or False. The baby born of a diabetic mother

a) The baby is at High risk of hypoglycaemia and respiratory distress and should be nursed in a neonatal intensive care unit.
b) The blood glucose must be checked four- hourly
c) Although the baby may have a good birth weight, manage the baby as a premature baby
d) Feed the baby on demand
e) Prevent hypothermia

274. Answer True or False. PRE-ECLAMPSIA is a syndrome characterised by:

a) High blood pressure
b) Oedema of abdomen, sacral region, puffy face, ankles and extending up the legs, swollen hands and fingers, swollen labia
c) Proteinuria.
d) Common in primiparous women
e) Affects short women only

275. In Pre-Eclampsia there is increased resistance in the arterioles due to vasospasm affecting mostly the brain, liver and kidneys. Which of the statements below are true?

a) Pre-eclampsia is common in the second trimester and rare before 24 weeks
b) Pre-eclampsia is associated with multiple pregnancy, diabetes, hydatidiform mole and essential hypertension.
c) It is important to monitor renal function of women with pre-eclampsia
d) The midwife must always record the blood pressure, test the urine for protein and record the presence of oedema.
e) Women with pre-eclampsia always develop eclampsia.

276. Which of the maternal conditions below are complications of pre-eclampsia?

a) Eclampsia
b) Renal failure
c) Abruption Placenta and haemorrhage
d) Cerebral haemorrhage and stroke
e) Premature labour

277. Which of the following are complications of pre-eclampsia on the Fetus?

a) Intra-uterine growth retardation
b) Prematurity
c) Light for dates
d) Intrauterine death
e) Neonatal death

278. Pregnancy induced hypertension has dangers to both the mother and the fetus. How should a midwife manage a client with PIH?

  a) The midwife must refer all clients with pre-eclampsia for management by specialist
  b) Clients with PIH must be monitored closely for blood pressure and fetal heart monitoring
  c) The midwife must advise the client on rest and monitoring fetal movements
  d) Monitor weight gain, oedema and protein in urine
  e) Let the client eat what she wants.

279. Answer True or False about care of a woman with PIH

  a) The client must have Drug therapy to include sedatives especially at night, Antihypertensive drugs and diuretics
  b) It may be necessary to admit the woman for blood pressure monitoring, fetal heart monitoring and renal function monitoring.
  c) Induction of labour can be done to deliver the woman before 37 weeks to prevent fetal loss.
  d) Any signs of fetal distress, rise in blood pressure and poor kidney function call for emergency caesarean section.
  e) After the woman is delivered, she is in less danger.

280. Answer True or False. Fetal monitoring in PIH includes

  a) Continuous or 4hourly fetal heart rate monitoring where the client is admitted in hospital
  b) Ultra sound fetal growth monitoring
  c) Hormonal assays for feto-placental function tests
  d) Amniocentesis for lung maturity test before emergency induction.
  e) Fetal movement chart

281. Which statements are true about management of Pregnancy Induced Hypertension,

  a) Induction of labour is done when hypertension and proteinuria persists

  b) Epidural anaesthesia is ideal as it reduces blood pressure

  c) The second stage of labour should be assisted

  d) The third stage of labour must be actively managed.

  e) Delivery of the baby is always at term

282. Which statements are true about management of a client who goes into an eclamptic fit?

a) Place client in a coma position and prepare for Caesarean Section
b) Infuse with IV fluids, with IV hypotensive drugs and anti-convulsive drugs according to local policy protocol
c) Check blood pressure and pulse every 10-15 minutes
d) Continuous fetal heart monitoring or every 10-15 minutes
e) Check for vaginal bleeding, cervical dilatation, state of membranes and liqour

283. Which of the statements below are true about multiple pregnancy?

a) Multiple pregnancy can occur from simultaneous fertilization of two or more ova by two or more spermatozoa
b) Dizygotic multiple pregnancy means one sperm fertilizes several ova
c) The ova may come from the same or different ovaries.
d) Each fetus is always in a separate sac has its own placenta.
e) The sex of the babies is always the same.

284. Identical twins are a result of division of a single fertilized ovum.

a) Monozygotic twins are also known as uni-ovular twins.
b) Monozygotic twins arise from equal division of the ovum at the inner cell mass stage.
c) The fetuses have a single placenta and one chorion but each fetus has its own amniotic sac.
d) Fetus papyraceous occurs when one of the multiple fetuses becomes dehydrated and dies in utero
e) Dizygotic twins are more common in families with twins, in older women and multigravid women.

285. Diagnosis of multiple pregnancy

a) The abdomen is larger than dates
b) The girth of the abdomen and size of the uterus is greater than expected
c) Multiple fetal movements can be seen
d) There are many fetal parts on palpation
e) More than one small fetal heads can be palpated

286. The complications of multiple pregnancy are:

a) Anaemia is more commonin multiple pregnancy than in a single pregnancy
b) Polyhydramnios is more likely in multiple pregnancy
c) Women with multiple pregnancy are prone to Eclampsia
d) Premature labour and Low birth weight are common
e) Locked twins and conjoined twins can occur

287. Which statements are true about the fetal skull?

a) The **Vault** of the fetal skull is made up of five bones
b) The two parietal bones are on the lateral sides of the skull
c) Two frontal bones are on the front of the skull
d) One occiput is on the back of the skull
e) There are Fourteen fused face bones.

288. Which of the following statements are true about the sutures of the fetal skull?

a) The two frontal bones are separated by the frontal suture
b) The saggital suture separates the 2 parietal bones
c) The frontal suture separates the frontal bone and the parietal bones
d) The lambdoidal suture separates the parietal bones and the occiput.
e) All sutures close by six weeks post delivery

289. Answer True or False about the sutures of the fetal skull

a) The posterior fontanelle or lambda is one finger wide.
b) The saggital suture, coronal sutures and the frontal suture meet at the bregma or anterior fontanelle.
c) Sutures overlap in labour in a process called moulding.
d) The bregma is diamond shaped
e) In post term babies all sutures are closed before delivery

300. Which statements are true about fetal skull moulding?

a) Excessive moulding can occur in premature babies
b) Excessive moulding may cause brain damage
c) Excessive moulding may cause tearing of the periosteum from the skull bones
d) In moulding the parietal bones glide over each other
e) A post term skull moulds better than a premature skull.

301. Which are the True Landmarks of the Fetal Skull?

a) Occipital Eminence
b) Parietal Eminence
c) The Bregma or anterior fontanelle
d) The Mentum or chin
e) The fourteen fused facial bones

302. How wide are the following presenting Diameters of the Fetal Skull?

a) Vertex Presentation or well flexed head.
b) After Coming head of breech(ACH)
c) Fully Extended Head or Face Presentation.
d) Face to Pubes
e) Brow Presentation.

303. During labour which engaging diameters of the fetal skull will be problematic?

a) Mento-Vertical or Brow presentation
b) Occipito- Frontal or Face to Pubes
c) Sub-Mento Bregmatic or Face presentation
d) Sub-Occipito Frontal
e) Sub-Occipito Bregmatic

304.TRUE or FALSE? The Pelvic Joints are:

a) 2 sacro-iliac joints
b) The symphysis pubis
c) Sacro-coccygeal joint
d) Th lumbar-sacral joint
e) The great trochanteric joint

305.Which of the following is true of the Pelvic ligaments?

a) Sacro-iliac ligaments bind the sacrum and ilium at the sacro-iliac joint
b) The inter-pubic ligaments are the strongest in the body
c) The sacro-tuberous ligament stretches from the sacrum to the ischial tuberosity
d) The sacro-spinous ligament between the sacrum and the spine of the ischium form the posterior wall of the pelvic outlet.
e) The lumbar-sacral ligaments bind the spine to the pelvis

306. Name three characteristics of each of the 4 types of pelves below

a) Gynaecoid pelvis
b) Android pelvis
c) Anthropoid pelvis
d) Platypelloid pelvis
e) Rachitic pelvis

307. What are the measurements of the gynaecoid pelvis?

a) The antero-posterior diameter of the brim is measured from-----------to-------- and is ----------cm. long
b) The oblique diameter of the brim is measured from-----------to-----------and is ----cm long.
c) The transverse diameter is measured from-------------- to--------------------and is---------cm long
d) The anatomical conjugate is measured from-------------to-------- and is ---cm.
e) The obstetric conjugate is measured from---------to------and is--------cm.

308. What is the significance of the following structures of the female pelvis?

a) The ischial spines
b) The bi-spinous diameter
c) The coccyx
d) The sacral promontory
e) The sacrum

309. Which type of female pelvis is described below?

a) A flat pelvis with a kidney shaped brim. It has a narrow antero-posterior diameter and the transverse diameter is wide. The sacrum is pushed forwards. Diameters of the brim, cavity and outlet are reduced.

b) The brim is round except where the promontory of the sacrum projects inwards, the outlet is diamond shaped.

c) The brim is heart shaped. The cavity is deep, and the outlet narrow like a funnel. The ischial spines are prominent.

d) Posterior positions are common. Deep transverse arrest of the head may occur

e) The brim is oval. The transverse diameter is reduced, less that the antero-posterior diameter. In labour the head may engage with occiput anterior but will not rotate.

310. Which are the True characteristics of labour pain?

a) Pain starts from the fundus of the uterus and moves down like a wave to sink in the groins and increases in intensity

b) Erratic irregular pain

c) Reduced time in between the pangs of pain until pain comes every 5-10 minutes and lasts up to fifty seconds.

d) Backache, a flame- like pain that intensifies on the small of the back and comes simultaneously with abdominal contraction.

e) Pain on passing urine

311. What advice would you give a pregnant woman if she complains of

leg cramps

a) Elevate your feet on a stool as you sit.
b) Drink a lot of milk to increase your calcium levels
c) Engage in regular exercise
d) Dorsiflex the foot of the affected leg
e) Lie on your left side to relieve pressure of the uterus on leg nerves

312. Which of the following are signs of pressure symptoms in pregnancy?

a) Ankle oedema
b) Breast tenderness
c) Heartburn
d) Haemorrhoids
e) Backache

313. An 18year old pregnant woman tells you she thinks she is in labour.

Which of the following suggest the onset of labour?

a) Abdominal pain
b) Rupture of the membranes
c) Observation of show
d) Backache
e) Frequency of micturition

314. What information can be obtained by doing a Vaginal examination?

a) The state of the vulva, sores, discharge, haemorrhoids, swelling
b) Cervical effacement or shortening can be established
c) Cervical dilatation
d) The adequacy of the pelvic cavity and outlet can be assessed
e) The presenting part of the fetus can be ascertained

315. What are the indications for vaginal examination in established labour?

a) To exclude cord presentation and cord prolapse
b) To determine descent of the presenting part
c) To assess the state of membranes and the type of liquor or vaginal discharge
d) To assess the degree of moulding and caput succedaneum
e) To diagnose the cause of delay in progress of labour

316. Which information is essential to record in established labour?

a) Fetal heart rate
b) Type of contractions.
c) State of membranes and colour of liquour
d) Analgesia and any other drugs given to the client
e) Client's blood pressure, temperature and respirations

317. Which of the following are Maternal causes of fetal hypoxia?

a) Anaemia,
b) Pre-clampsia and eclampsia
c) Heart disease especially Grade 3 and 4,
d) Weak to mild contractions
e) Placental dysfunction eg. Abruption placentae

318. Which of the following are true causes of fetal hypoxia?

a) Cord round the neck or limb
b) True knots in the cord
c) Placental infarcts
d) Cord presentation
e) Prolonged labour

319. Which of these statements are indicative of fetal distress?

a) Fetal tarchycardia or heart rate of more than 160 beats
b) Fetal brardycardia or heart rate below 110
c) Meconeum in the liquour
d) Fetal heart rate fluctuations during and after contractions
e) Sluggish fetal movements during labour.

320. How would you manage fetal distress in first stage of labour?

a) Communicate with client about observations
b) Nurse patient in an upright position
c) Infuse the client with IVI Dextrose 10%
d) If on oxytocin, stop the infusion
e) Give oxygen and prepare for Caesarean section

321. You discover fetal distress in a primiparous woman during the second stage of labour. What actions should you take?

a) Perform an episiotomy to quicken delivery
b) Prepare for forceps delivery or vacuum extraction depending on available expertise
c) Prepare for fetal resuscitation
d) Tell the client to quickly push the baby out
e) Give oxygen to the mother

322. If a woman opts for the natural methods of pain relief in labour, which methods can a midwife offer?

a) A woman can take a warm shower or soak herself in a warm bath as she labours.
b) A woman can take deep breaths with contractions.
c) A woman can adopt positions that shorten labour.
d) Barbiturates and tranquilizers can be given in early labour.
e) Massage can be offered.

323. Which of the following are the effects of Pethidine and Morphine on the mother and fetus?

a) Maternal drowsiness
b) They cause poor maternal effort in the second stage of labour.
c) They cause fetal distress
d) They increase the need for fetal resuscitation.
e) They are safe drugs that can be given any time during labour.

324. Which statements are true about Inhalation Analgesia?

a) It is most useful in the late first stage and second stage of labour
b) It must be used before a contraction.
c) It requires an anaesthetist to administer it.
d) The client must be familiar with deep breathing technique.
e) It has no residual effect on the infant.

325. Which statements are True about Epidural anaesthesia in labor?

a) It enables the woman to be a full participant in her labour process
b) It allows all procedures to be done without the need for additional anaesthesia.
c) It enables a painless labour and operative delivery without affecting consciousness
d) It does not cross the placental barrier to affect the fetus
e) It causes drowsiness

326. Which of the following statements are true of Epidural anaesthesia?

a) It requires an anaesthetist to administer it making it accessible to a small percentage of women.
b) It lowers blood pressure
c) The client is confined to bed
d) The client requires catheterization
e) It affects maternal effort in the second stage of labour increasing the need for assisted delivery such as forceps delivery

327. Fill in the gaps in mechanism of vertex presentation

a) With increased contractions, the head is flexed and descent takes place with increasing -----------------------.
b) The occiput reaches the pelvic floor first and rotates 1/8 of a circle forwards to become -----------
c) The occiput escapes under the --------------------in a process called-----------
d) The sinciput, face and chin sweep the perineum and the head is born by a movement of---------------.
e) The anterior shoulder reaches the pelvic floor first and rotates 1/8 of a circle forwards at the same time as there is external rotation of the head.
The rest of the body is delivered by a movement of ---------------.

328. Place these stages of the mechanism of vertex presentation sequentially.

a) Restitution
b) Internal rotation of shoulders
c) Crowning
d) Internal rotation of head
e) Flexion

329. In Breech presentation

a) There are three classifications of breech presentation namely, Breech with extended legs, Breech with flexed legs, Footling and knee presentations
b) Breech presentation is associated with big babies and premature babies
c) Breech is associated with a long cord.
d) The placenta is usually situated in the fundus of the uterus
e) In multiple pregnancy, one fetus may adopt a breech position

330. In the diagnosis of a breech by palpation:

a) The head can be palpated in the fundus
b) The lie is longitudinal
c) There is a large irregular soft mass on pelvic palpation and Pawlick's grip
d) The fetal heart is heard above the umbilicus
e) Fetal parts can be palpated all over the abdomen

331. Which statements are true about the Mechanism of Breech Delivery?

a) Engagement of the breech occurs in the oblique or transverse diameter of the pelvic brim
b) The bi-trochanteric diameter lies in the antero-posterior diameter of the pelvic outlet.
c) The anterior buttock appears at the vulva by lateral flexion of the trunk
d) The buttocks are born while the shoulders adjust to engage in the transverse diameter of the brim.
e) When shoulders reach the pelvic floor, they undergo internal rotation so that the bisachromial diameter lies in the antero-posterior diameter of the pelvic outlet.

332. TRUE or FALSE? In Management of labour in breech presentation a midwife must:

a) Always deliver the breech
b) Refer all breech presentation to hospital with facility for Caesarean Section.
c) Confirm presentation through a vaginal examination
d) Exclude cord prolapsed when membranes rupture
e) Manage labour like any normal labour

333. TRUE or FALSE? In the delivery of a breech presentation:

a) An episiotomy must always be done as the buttocks distend the vulva
b) Allow the natural process of delivery where possible.
c) Slight traction can be applied to deliver buttocks.
d) Extended legs of breech can be released by applying pressure on the popliteal fossa
e) The loop of the cord is gently brought down to prevent traction on the cord which causes fetal distress.

334. Which statements are FALSE about Breech Delivery?

a) The Lovset manoeuvre delivers shoulders by rotating the body of the baby 180 degrees.
b) Always maintain full flexion of the head.
c) You should never touch the breech, it delivers itself.
d) The head is always delivered with slight supra-pubic pressure
e) **The Mauriceau–Smellie-Veit technique** is an alternative method for delivery of the after coming head of breech.

335. TRUE/FALSE. Fetal Complications of breech delivery are:

a) Cord prolapse
b) Fetal distress
c) Fractures of limbs
d) Abruptio placenta
e) Impacted shoulders

336. Which events are likely in breech delivery?

a) Arrest of aftercoming head
b) Brain injury
c) Nerve injury
d) Precipitate labour
e) Stillbirth or neonatal death

337. Which are the complications associated with Breech delivery?

a) Extensive Cervical, vaginal and perineal tears
b) Haemorrhage
c) Maternal dehydration
d) Ascending Infection
e) Symphyseal rupture

338. Which statements are true about the positions adopted in labour?

a) The fetus can descend into the pelvis assisted by gravity if the client maintains an upright position.
b) The fetus follows the natural Curve of Carus, into the pelvis.
c) Lying in bed slows down labour
d) Leaning against one's partner is ideal for back massage and enables the partner to participate actively in the events of labour
e) Walking about should be permissible even in early rapture of membranes with a high head

339. TRUE/FALSE. In the first stage of labour a woman can:

a) Sit in a firm chair with a firm straight back.
b) Squat for long or short periods depending.
c) Kneel and leaning on cushions or pillows
d) Sit in a warm tub of water.
e) Practice yoga

340.Which are the Advantages of upright positions in labour?

a) The labouring woman's partner can assist with back massage.
b) Women experience less painful labour f.
c) The fetus has a good supply of oxygen throughout the first stage of labour.
d) The uterine muscles contract more efficiently.
e) The cervical dilation is faster as the presenting part applies to the cervix better.

341. Which of the following are diagnostic of the onset of the second stage of labour?

a) Full dilatation of the cervix
b) Client vomiting
c) Expulsive strong contractions lasting 60-90 seconds 3-5minute intervals
d) The presenting part lies on the perineum
e) Maternal dehydration

342. During the second stage of labour, which of the following events should cause concern?

a) Fetal heart beat of 140 beats per minute?
b) Thick meconeum?
c) Bloody vaginal discharge?
d) Clear liquor?
e) Maternal sweating?

343. In second stage of labour, when do you take the following action?

a) Infuse the client with 5%Dextrose infusion and give oxygen
b) Prepare for assisted delivery- vacuum extraction, forceps delivery to quicken delivery.
c) Prepare for emergency Caesarean Section
d) Call a paediatrician
e) Communicate with the labouring woman?

344.The following is true of upright Delivery Positions

a) The baby descends by gravity.
b) The client is more comfortable than lying down.
c) The second stage of labour is shortened.
d) Perineal tears and Post- partum haemorrhage are minimal
e) The newly born baby is stressed increasing the need for neonatal resuscitation.

345.Episiotomy is a surgical incision made on the perineum during the perineal phase of labour. Which statements are true about episiotomy?

a) It prevents ragged perineal tears
b) It protects rectal muscle
c) It prevents pressure and injury to fetal head
d) It enables quick delivery of the baby.
e) It is elective for all primiparous women.

346. True or False? When performing an episiotomy procedure

a) Two fingers are placed between presenting part and perineal muscle to prevent injury to the fetus
b) 5-10mls of lignocaine are injected into perineal muscle in a fan-like manner
c) Incision is made with a contraction
d) For best healing results the episiotomy is sutured in one layer.
e) The perineum can be sutured within twenty-four hours.

347. TRUE/FALSE. The following precautions must be taken

during the perineal stage of labor

a) As the head distends the perineum, the tightness of the perineal muscles must be assessed.
b) As the head escapes through the vagina feel for the cord around the neck.
c) Allow for restitution to take place
d) Clear the airways
e) Give the baby Vit. K1 on the upper arm

348. True or False? Active management of the third stage of labour

involves the following:

a) Give syntometrine with delivery of the anterior shoulder
b) Deliver the placenta by cord traction
c) Allow the placenta to fall out of the birth canal
d) Squeeze the fundus to expel the placenta.
e) Collect cord blood.

349. TRUE/FALSE The following statements are true about the third stage of labour

a) Placenta separates from maternal uterine wall within three minutes of the birth of the child
b) The raw placental area is about 7.5cm wide post delivery
c) Myometrial function is to control haemorrhage post- delivery.
d) Post-partum haemorrhage occurs mostly in primiparous women
e) The height of fundus should be below the umbilicus after delivery

350.TRUE/FALSE. The following are signs of placental separation

a) A gush of blood may escape through the vagina
b) The cord lengthens
c) The height of the fundus rises
d) The contractions cease
e) The maternal blood pressure rises

351.Which statements are true?

a) In the Shultze method of placental delivery, the placenta slips through a hole in the membranes and the fetal side appears at the vulva with the membranes trailing behind like an inverted umbrella.
b) The Matthews Duncan method of placental delivery,the placenta slides down sideways with the lateral border first like a button through a button hole. The maternal side is exposed and blood escapes
c) The umbilical cord Extends from the fetal umbilicus to the fetal surface of the placenta.
d) The umbilical cord is composed of connective tissue and Wharton's jelly covered by the amnion.
e) The umbilical cord has two arteries, an extension of the hypogastric arteries.

352. TRUE or FALSE?

a) Umbilical arteries carry impure blood to the placenta
b) A single artery is associated with other congenital abnormalities of the fetus.
c) Umbilical vein contains pure blood from the placenta to the fetus.
d) Hold the placenta by the cord so that the membranes hang like an inverted umbrella
e) The average length of the umbilical cord should be about 56cms.

353. During the examination of the placenta, what observations

   must a midwife make?

a) Presence of true knots which could be the cause of fetal distress and still birth
b) Count the blood vessels in the cord
c) Note any missing portions of the membranes as these are a source of post-partum haemorrhage
d) Note any blood vessels running to the edge of the membranes suggesting a succenturiate lobe which may cause haemorrhage and infection
e) Note any holes in the membranes suggestive of a missing lobe

354. Before disposal of the placenta, a midwife must:

a) Expose the maternal side and clean it with swab collecting any

   retro-placental clot and add to blood loss

b) Inspect the cotyledons- absence of one suggestive of retained lobe, a source of post- partum haemorrhage
c) Take note of placental infarcts
d) Weigh the placenta-it should be 1/6 of the baby's weight.
e) Collect cord blood

355. Before transferring the client to the postnatal ward:

a) Inspect genital tract in good light for tears
b) Repair the episiotomy and tears
c) Check blood pressure and pulse
d) Check height of fundus if high rub up a contraction to expel clots
e) Check if infant is in good condition

356. Obstructed Labour means there is no advance of presenting part in the presence of good contractions. Are the following causes True or False?

a) The passenger

b) The Powers

c) The passages

d) Poor maternal effort

e) Early bearing down

357. True or False? Obstructed labour may be due to

a) Contracted pelvis
b) Transverse lie in a preterm labour
c) Tumours eg fibroids
d) Macrosomia
e) Fetal abnormalities e.g.hydrocephalus, double headed monster, conjoined twins

358.True or False? Obstructed labour at the inlet may be due to:

a) Android pelvis

b) Weak contractions

c) Scoliosis

d) Gross fetal abnormalities

e) Compound presentation

359. True or False? Mid-cavity obstruction can be due to:

a) Prominent ischial spines

b) Footling breech

c) Shoulder dystocia

d) Anencephaly

e) Multiple pregnancy

360.True or False? Obstruction at the outlet can be due to:

a) Tight perineal muscles

b) Rachitic pelvis

c) Impacted shoulders

d) Brow presentation

e) Poor maternal effort

361. Which statements are true of the signs of obstructed

labour?

a) The presenting part remains floating above the inlet despite good contractions
b) The cervix dilates slowly and hangs loosely like an empty sleeve
c) Membranes remain intact
d) The uterus moulds around the fetus and does not relax between contractions
e) The presenting part is wedged or stuck in the pelvis

362. You are observing a woman in labour, what would the following features mean to you?

a) Excessive moulding occurs
b) A large caput forms
c) Contractions cease for a while and recommence with renewed vigour
d) Bandl's ring seen around the umbilicus
e) Maternal ketosis
f) Meconium stained liquor

363. What are the dangers of Obstructed labour to the mother?

a) Rupture of uterus
b) Haemorrhage
c) Loss of memory
d) Fistula
e) Rupture of the bladder
f) Death

364. What are the dangers of obstructed labour to the fetus?

a) Fetal hypoxia
b) Intracranial haemorrhage
c) Cerebral palsy
d) Stillbirth
e) Neonatal death

365. What prophylaxis measures can a midwife put in place in preventing obstructed labour?

a) Early diagnosis of fetal abnormalities
b) Careful monitoring during labour to make early diagnosis of obstruction
c) Refer to obstetrician all women likely to have obstructed labour
d) Encourage women to seek professional care when in labour
e) Relax, let nature take its course

366. What are the causes of rupture of the uterus?

a) Obstructed labour
b) Trauma during difficult deliveries e.g. shoulder dystocia, after coming head of breech
c) High doses of oxytocin
d) Weak caesarean scar
e) Uncomfortable position in labour

367. Which of the following are not dangers of Ruptured Uterus?

a) Severe haemorrhage that may lead to maternal death
b) Sheehan's syndrome
c) Fetal loss
d) Secondary infertility
e) Weak bladder

368. Which of the following are warning signs of uterine rupture?

a) Tonic contractions
b) Bandl's ring
c) Signs of internal haemorrhage such as rapid pulse, restlessness, low blood pressure, sighing respirations
d) Very tender lower abdomen
e) Very high blood pressure

369. Which of the following are not signs of actual rupture of the uterus?

a) The woman may feel that something has given way
b) The woman has meconium stained liquor
c) The fetus can be palpated under the abdominal wall
d) The woman may complain of shoulder pain a sign of blood in the peritoneum
e) The uterus can be felt as a separate mass in the abdomen

370. Which of the following are true of rupture of a weak caesarean scar?

a) Rupture may be due to poor healing or pregnancy soon after previous caesarean section
b) Rupture of the scar usually occurs during the last weeks of pregnancy
c) 'Silent rupture' may occur in the first stage of labour
d) Rupture is sudden and tears across the uterine body
e) Client complains of intermittent abdominal pain
f) Client has severe abdominal pain and heavy vaginal bleeding

371. How do you manage clients with previous caesarean deliveries?

a) All clients with previous Caesarean deliveries must have a hospital delivery
b) Oxytocin should not be used on clients with previous caesarean deliveries
c) Abdominal palpation in clients with previous caesarean section must not be done
d) Complaints of abdominal pain or pain over the scar must be taken seriously
e) Observe closely for signs of shock and vaginal bleeding

372. Which statements are true general principles of managing a pregnant woman

a) Aim at making early diagnosis of fetal mal-presentation and refer
b) Check the blood pressure and test the urine in the second trimester.
c) Provide factual information about the progress of her pregnancy
d) Provide relevant phase related health education
e) Prepare the woman for induction of labour

373. Which of the following are likely causes of intrauterine death?

a) Infections such as HIV
b) Pre-eclampsia, antepartum haemorrhage
c) Diabetes, Rhesus incompatibility
d) Poor diet
e) Placental infarcts

374. Which of the following are signs of intra-uterine fetal death?

a) Abscence of fetal heart beat
b) The mother does not feel fetal movements
c) There is no uterine growth
d) The height of fundus is large for dates
e) Ultrasound scan shows Spalding's sign- gross overlapping of fetal skull bones

375. What would be your diagnosis if

a) On xray intra-fetal gas or bubbles of air can be seen in the lungs and heart of fetus?
b) On xray, the thoracic cage of the fetus is collapsed?
c) There is hyper-flexion of the spine with abnormal fetal attitudes?
d) On palpation, there are two round masses?
e) The abdomen feels doughy and broad?

376. An ultra-sound scan reveals Spalding's sign in a woman who is 32 weeks pregnant. What is the management?

a) Inform the couple of findings and likely management
b) Labour is induced
c) The fetus is already dead, so wait for nature to take its course
d) Do an amniocentesis
e) Offer Family planning advice

377. True or False? The causes of Fresh Stillbirth are:

a) Hypoxia due to Placental insufficiency in pre-eclampsia, diabetes, renal disease, post maturity, true knots in the cord.
b) Abruption placenta
c) Smoking in the mother
d) Uterine inertia
e) Shoulder dystocia

378. Post maturity is when pregnancy goes beyond 42 weeks 297 How do you manage a case of post maturity?

a) Ascertain pregnancy dates.

b) Induce labour

c) Will need an episiotomy and assisted delivery

d) Delivery must always by Caesarean section

379. What are the risks of post maturity?

a) Stillbirth
b) Placental insufficiency is common
c) Cervical, vaginal and perineal tears
d) The mother is tired
e) Birth injuries are common

380. What are the features of a post mature baby?

a) Has hard skull bones, small fontanelles and narrow sutures
b) The skin is dry and peeling off
c) There is no subcutaneous fat
d) Nails are long
   a) The baby does not cry on delivery

381. Which situations call for the need for a Caesarean Section?

a) Gross fetal abnormalities e.g.hydrocephalus

b) Obstructed labour

c) Locked twins

d) In severe fetal distress.

f) False labour.

382. Which Maternal conditions require a caesarean section?

a) Severe Pre-eclampsia and eclampsia.
b) Abnormal uterine action.
c) Contracted pelvis
d) Cephalo pelvic disproportion
e) Previous Caesarean section

383. Caesarean Section can be done to save a baby in the following conditions .

a) Macrosomia such as in diabetes and potential diabetes
b) Transverse Lie.
c) Compound Presentation
d) A small baby as in premature labour
e) Shoulder dystocia

384. The following conditions would require referral to an obstetrician. Which of these would be more urgent?

a) Abnormal fetus eg hydrocephalus, suspected conjoined twins at 36 weeks
b) Locked twins in labour
c) Retained twin with normal heart beat
d) Fetal tarchycardia or bradycardia at 8cm of cervical dilation in a primiparous woman
e) Cord Prolapse
f) Cord presentation.

385. Which statements are true of Lower segment caesarean section or Pfannestiel incision

a) It is transverse just above the symphysis pubis

b) It heals well and the scar may not be obvious

c) Makes early ambulation easy

d) Does not interfere with sitting and breast feeding

e) May heal quickly in obese women

386. Which is true of Classical Caesarean section

a) The incision extends from above the symphysis pubis to the umbilicus or just above
b) Uterine incision extends to the upper segment
c) It is uncomfortable when client tries to sit and inhibits breastfeeding
d) It is slow in healing and limits client's activity post delivery
e) It is prone to wound dehiscence

387. What are the important aspects of care for a woman after

Caesarean Section?

a) Let the client eat as much of what she wants as possible
b) Look out for bleeding from wound and signs of internal haemorrhage
c) Pain relief must be given according to client's needs
d) The client must be assisted in finding comfortable breast- feeding positions
e) Encourage mobility to prevent deep vein thrombosis and hypostatic pneumonia

388. Which of these statements would constitute good advice to a primiparous client after Caesarean Section?

a) Following an epidural anaesthesia, she must engage in leg movements to prevent deep vein thrombosis.
b) To prevent chest complications, she must engage in deep breathing exercises as soon as possible.
c) Avoid strenuous activity and allow the body time to recover and the wound time to heal.
d) A nutritious diet rich in fruit and vegetables.
e) Avoid a pregnancy until the doctor advises.

389.Which statements are true about Post- Partum Hemorrhage?

a) Hemorrhage is one of the leading causes of maternal mortality in the world
b) Blood loss of more than 600mls after delivery of a baby is termed Primary post-partum hemorrhage.
c) Bleeding in the first 24 hours post-delivery is due to failure of effective uterine contraction.
d) Uterine atony is common in multiparous women, multiple pregnancy, hydatidiform mole, fibroids, prolonged labor, following general anesthesia

390.The following types of haemorrhage must be treated as

emergency. TRUE or FALSE?

a) Retention of placental tissue
b) Abruption placenta and placenta praevia
c) Clotting defects such as hypo-fibrinogenaemia and low platlets and other blood discrasias
d) Ruptured uterus or torn cervix or vaginal wall lacerations
e) Heavy menses

391. Secondary post- partum haemorrhage occurs after 24hours.Which of these are causes of secondary Post- Partum Hemorrhage? TRUE or FALSE?

a) Retained membranes or placental cotyledon
b) Dislogded clot
c) Infection such as myometritis
d) Onset of choriocarcinoma
e) Onset of menses

392. Which are True Signs of severe blood loss?

a) Restlessness followed by severe weakness
b) Rapid thready pulse and low blood pressure.
c) Polyuria
d) Breathlessness and sighing respirations
e) The skin becomes pale, dusky, cold and clammy

393. Which of these are true Principles of managing hemorrhage

a) Replace lost fluids through an intravenous line.
b) Quickly identify source of the haemorrhage and manage accordingly
   In abortion evacuation of uterus to remove retained products of conception
   and an oxytocic drug may be needed
c) Infection must be treated with antibiotics
d) Give nothing by mouth

394. Which simple measures can a midwife take to prevent loss of lives through haemorrhage?

a) Immediate transfer of women to facilities with adequate resources for resuscitation.
b) Close monitoring of vaginal bleeding Pad checks should be done hourly in the first two hours post-delivery, then two hourly for four hours then four hourly thereafter.
c) Monitoring women for signs of internal haemorrhage through blood pressure and pulse every half hour post delivery
d) Fundal Height measurement. Fundal height may rise where there is internal bleeding due to atony of the uterus.
e) Weighing the client daily

395. Which of the following clients are likely to have postpartum haemorrhage?

a) Primiparous clients
b) Clients who have had difficult prolonged labour,
c) Clients who have had multiple deliveries
d) Clients who have had surgical deliveries.
e) Clients who had polyhydramnios

396. Which statements are true about events post- delivery,

a) The consistency of the contracted uterus must feel like a tennis ball.

b) A soft boggy or dough-like uterus is a sign of poor contraction of

   the uterus

c) The height of the fundus is below the umbilicus and should continue   to decrease until the uterus is no longer palpable around fourteen days post-delivery.

d) The fundal height should be measured on a day-to-day basis and should decrease by approximately one centimetre a day post- delivery.

e) Sudden haemorrhage is due to raised fluid intake

397. If a primiparous woman who has had an episiotomy complains of perineal discomfort. How can you assist her?

a) Check for perineal lacerations and give mild analgesics

b) Advise client to wash the perineum clean with each change of sanitary towel or every two hours to avoid odours and to promote healing.

c) Check episiotomy for haematoma, swelling and state of sutures

d) Advise on perineal muscle exercise

e) Advise on cold compress

398. How can a midwife help to prevent anaemia among her clients?

a) All women should have their haemoglobin checked before discharge from the postnatal ward.

b) The midwife must exclude anaemia in women who are lethargic, frail and tend to have a slow recovery post- delivery.

c) The midwife must provide health education on diet rich in iron

d) The midwife must advise on family planning to space pregnancies

e) The midwife must encourage routine check of clients haemoglobin periodically.

399. Which statements are true about prevention of bladder complications post delivery?

a) Encourage client to empty her bladder two hourly to prevent over-distension of the bladder.
b) Encourage client to take plenty of fluids to encourage the bladder to empty frequently by so doing regaining its tone.
c) Observe for hesitancy to empty the bladder and retention of urine..
d) Test for urinary tract infection if client has dysuria
e) Urine retention post-delivery is associated with damage to nerves and hypotonic pelvic musculature. The midwife can encourage her clients to engage in pelvic floor muscle exercises

400. Which statements are true about thrombo-embolic conditions post-delivery?

a) Clients who are bed-ridden or stay in bed for long periods can get thromboembolic complications
b) Any woman can get thrombo-embolic complications.
c) One of the causes of a high temperature post delivery could be thromboembolic complication
d) Early ambulation and passive limb movements, deep breathing in bed prevents thrombo-embolic complications
e) Suspect thrombo-embolic complications in a client with pain and severe heat in the lower limbs

401. Which statements are true about some of the measures that a midwife can take to prevent neonatal morbidity and mortality at birth?

a) Ensure that the baby cries at birth to establish good respiration and circulation. A good cry expands the lungs and establishes good respiration and normal circulation.
b) Administer oxygen by face mask if there are signs of cyanosis
c) Wipe baby dry and drape warmly to prevent hypothermia.
d) A quick examination of the new-born must be done as soon as the baby is born to diagnose obvious abnormalities that may expose the baby to morbidity and mortality.
e) Encourage breast feeding immediately

402. Examination of the newborn must be done after delivery and within 24hours to identify abnormalities. What features does a midwife look for on the baby's head?

a) The size and shape of the head to exclude hydrocephalus.
b) Microcephaly in which the head is small for the body
c) Anencephally where the cerebellum is absent
d) Cephalohaematoma
e) Caput succedenium

403.In the event of a midwife diagnosing a possible hydrocephaly.

The management would include:

a) The midwife must do a careful palpation to make an early diagnosis
b) Refer for verification of diagnosis if unsure
c) In early diagnosis, a therapeutic abortion is done
d) In late diagnosis, a caesarean section is performed
e) In obstructed labour a craniotomy is done

404. Which features pertain to an encephalocele and which ones pertain to a meningocele?

a) It is a tumour of the brain covered with meninges and protrudes through

the lambda or the sutures.

b) Depending on the size it may obstruct labour
c) Contains brain substance
d) Contains cerebro-spinal fluid
e) It is opaque
f) It does not fluctuate
g) Usually has a pedicle
h) Is fluctuant
i) Does not pulsate
j) Becomes tense when the baby cries
k) May rupture during labour otherwise it is corrected surgically

405. Which statements are true of an Anencephally?

a) It is a severe derformity common in female fetus in which the vault

of the skull and cerebellum are absent

b) It may be accompanied by spina bifida

c) Polyhydramnios is present in pregnancy

d) Increased levels of alphafetoproteins in amniotic fluid in

early pregnancy

e) Tendency for premature short labour

406. Which statements are true about Spina Bifida?

a) Spina Bifida is failure of the neural arches of the vertebrae to unite
b) Meninges and sometimes the spinal cord may protrude
c) Sometimes the structures are not covered with skin
d) The midwife can stitch the open wound before referral
e) There is no complication after wound closure

407. In which conditions should the midwife observe for trauma

and signs of intracranial injury in the first 24hours?

a) Baby born of a mother with contracted pelvis,
b) Large baby
c) Where the baby adopted an occipito-posterior position in labour
d) In breech delivery
e) Where there was Precipitate labour

408. In which conditions are the following birth injuries commonly found?

a) Dislocated hip
b) Fractured clavicle
c) Torticollis
d) Erb's palsy
e) Cephalohaematoma

409. Which injuries are described below?
   a) It is due to pressure of the cervix on presenting part of the head
   b) The presenting part becomes congested and oedematous
   c) It may occur in prolonged labour such as occipito-posterior
   d) Excessive moulding Is present at birth

404. Which statements describe the features of Caput succedaneum

or Cephalhaematoma?
   a) Swelling on the fetal skull
   b) It is effusion of blood under the periosteum
   c) Caused by friction between the fetal skull and pelvis
   d) Excessive moulding Is present at birth
   e) Pits on pressure
   f) Grows larger as bleeding occurs
   g) May persist for two weeks or more
   h) It is firm and does not pit on pressure
   i) May cross a suture
   j) Reduces in size with time
   k) Should disappear within 36hours
   l) It is always unilateral
   m) Can be bilateral
   n) It occurs commonly in cephalopelvic disproportion
   o) It can occur in quick delivery of the head such as in precipitate labour and after coming head of breech
   p) Appears after 12hours of childbirth
   q) Does not cross a suture

405. In which situations are the following fractures of the newborn likely to occur?

   a) Fractured or indentations on the skull
   b) Fracture of the humerus
   c) Fractures of Femur
   d) Fracture of the spine
   e) Fractured wrist

406. Which statements are true of Facial palsy?

a) Common in forceps delivery where the 7th cranial nerve may be pinched during delivery of the head.
b) One side of the mouth droops and milk may dribble during feeding
c) The eye on the affected side remains open
d) Corrects itself after a few weeks
e) Requires surgery to correct it

407. TRUE or FALSE? When the neck is accidentally twisted in breech delivery and shoulder dystocia the baby may sustain the following injuries:

a) Erb's paralysis or waiter's tip arm
b) Injury to the brachial plexus under the clavicle.
c) Facial palsy.
d) Paralysis of the lower legs
e) Slipped disk

408. Which statements are true about diagnosis and management of a baby suspected of sustaining injury to internal organs?

a) The baby is likely to have been delivered by Caesarean section
b) The liver and spleen are usually bruised
c) Haemoglobin must be checked within 24 hours.
d) The baby turns grey, passes bloody stools or collapses soon after delivery
e) The abdominal girth increases hourly

409.The following statements are true of Cleft lip and palate

a) There is lack of union of the fronto-nasal palate.
b) A baby may have just a cleft lip or may have both cleft lip and palate
c) These deformities are rarely unilateral
d) Special feeding apparatus with palate plates can be used for feeding the baby.
e) Corrective surgery can be done as early as in a week

410. What features can lead you to suspect oesophageal atresia, duodenal atresia, hernia, and imperforate anus, exomphalos in a newly born baby?

a) A rectal thermometer cannot be passed
b) The baby frothes from the mouth and nostrils on first feed.
c) The baby has projectile vomiting
d) Baby has projectile vomiting of mucus is noted
e) Waves of peristalsis can be noted on the abdomen after feeds
f) Usually noticed after the first week
g) A fine nasogastric tube fails to go down.
h) The baby vomits milk followed by bile characterized by green vomitus
i) A swelling around the umbilicus noted after the umbilical cord has dropped off
j) The baby's abdomen distends gradually
k) The baby does not pass meconium.
l) On inspection there may be a dimple in the cleft of the buttocks
m) The abdominal contents are outside the abdominal wall.

411. TRUE or FALSE? Women are advised to desist from using off the counter drugs in the first trimester to prevent the following

a) Amelia or absence of arms in the fetus
b) Phocomelia or abscence of long bones in the fetus
c) Nausea and vomiting
d) Excessive weight gain
e) Abortion

412. The midwife must advise clients to avoid the following drugs in early pregnancy. TRUE or FALSE?

a) Phenobarbitone
b) Diazepam
c) Chloroquin
d) Chloromycetin
e) Penicillin

413.TRUE or FALSE? When prescribing drugs, a midwife must

a) Advise clients against use of off the counter drugs in pregnancy
b) Always ask women if they are pregnant.
c) Always ask women if they are breast- feeding
d) Ask women about their last menstrual period
e) Ask women about allergies

414. TRUE or FALSE? Club Foot or Talipes Equino Varus is

a) When a baby is born with a foot that is bent downwards and inwards
b) Talippes Equino Varus may be unilateral (one foot) or bilateral (both feet)
c) Associated with oligohydramnios and maternal tumours like fibroids
d) Always bilateral
e) Can be corrected by splinting, application of Plaster of Paris and surgery

415. TRUE or FALSE?. A baby born with

a) Talipes Calcaneo-Valgus has a foot turned outwards.
b) Achondroplasia has short limbs
c) Mongolism/ Down's syndrome (Trisomy 21) has an extra chromosome ; thus 47 chromosomes instead of 46
d) Mongolism is associated with maternal ageing and is significant in mothers over the age of 35
e) A baby with extra digits usually has another deformity

416.TRUE or FALSE.The following are Characteristics of mongolism

a) Small head with flat occiput
b) Low set ears
c) Upward slanting eyes
d) Small mouth and large tongue
e) Large nose

417.You have doing examination of a newly-born baby, which features would convince you that the baby has mongolism?

a) Short hands
b) An unbroken palmer crease from side to side (the simian crease)
c) A widely separated large toe from the rest of the toes
d) Large eyes
e) Hairy body

418. The baby's reaction to various tests must be checked to assess for alertness and normalcy in the baby. How do you check for:

a) The Rooting Reflex

b) The Walking /Stepping Reflex

c) Moro Reflex

d) The Grasp Reflex

e) Asymmetrical Tonic Neck Reflex?

419. What are you checking for in

a) Glabellar Reflex
b) Rooting reflex
c) Moro reflex
d) Percussion
e) Measuring the baby's head circumference?

420. In what order must the midwife working in a neonatal unit attend to the following neonates?

a) A on day old infant crying persistently with a sharp shrill voice
b) A 12hour infant with rib recession
c) A five- hour old infant with blue extremities
d) A 6-hour old large for dates infant of a diabetic mother sleeping quietly
e) A three- hour old infant with tarchycardia of180 beats per minute

421. The following statements are true of breast milk

a) Breast milk contains immune bodies to prevent infections in the baby.
b) Breast milk is nutritious with all food values in the correct proportions
c) Breast milk is 80%water
d) Breast feeding promotes close relationships between mother and baby
e) Breast milk has laxative property preventing constipation in the baby.

422. What infections are the following micro-organisms likely to cause in mother or baby?

  a) Clostridium Welchii

  b) Streptococcus B

  c) Clostridium tetani

  d) Staphylococcus

  e) Pneumococci

423. The midwife is caring for an Rh-negative mother who has delivered an Rh-positive infant. Which of the following statements are true?

  a) RhoGam is given to the infant to prevent development of antibodies
  b) RhoGam is given to the infant to supply the necessary antibodies
  c) RhoGam is given to the mother to prevent formation of antibodies against future Rh-positive infants
  d) RhoGam is given to the mother to encourage formation of antibodies against Rh-positive babies
  e) RhoGam should not be given at all

424. On postnatal domiciliary visits, a midwife finds a baby who is moderately jaundiced. What advice is appropriate to the mother?

  a) You must improve your diet.
  b) Breast-feed your baby for at least twenty minutes per breast three-hourly
  c) Drink a lot of nutritious fluids to improve lactation
  d) Ensure the umbilicus is clean
  e) That is what happens to all babies; your baby will be well.

425. What are the possible causes for the following observations in a new born infant?

  a) Frothing
  b) Regurgitation of feeds
  c) Cyanosis during breast feeding
  d) Facial muscle twitching
  e) Anuria

110

426. Which statements describe some of the symptoms a woman with fibroids may experience?

a) Constipation.

b) Hemorrhoids.

c) Heartburn

d) Varicose veins on the legs.

e) Frequency of micturition and dribbling of urine.

427. Which of the following are effects of Fibroids on Reproduction?

a) Abortion, and premature labor.

b) Excessive pain, uterine inertia, obstructed labor

c) Post- partum hemorrhage

d) High blood pressure

e) Dyspareunia

428. In management of fibroids, which of the following statements are true?

a) Fibroids identified during pregnancy are usually removed during delivery.
b) Myomectomy or removal of the fibroid is done where one is still young and would like to have babies.
c) It is important to ensure that one's female tubes are not blocked before myomectomy.
d) If one is over forty a hysterectomy (removal of the uterus) is advisable.
e) Fibroids almost always become cancerous

429. The following women are likely to have cancer of the cervix

a) Cancer of the cervix affects any woman of any race
b) Sexually active women are mostly affected
c) Women who have had a few pregnancies are likely to get cancer
d) Women who had early exposure to sexual activity
e) Women who have had only one sexual

430. Is it true that one can suspect cancer of the cervix or the female internal organs if:

a) One notices some bleeding after intercourse
b) One has abnormal bleeding that is not related to the monthly cycle
c) One experiences pain on sexual intercourse
d) One has lower abdominal pain that is not caused by anything notable.
e) One feels a lump or mass in the lower abdomen

431. What Health Education can be given a woman after Cone Biopsy?

a) Do not use tampons until the cervix is completely healed which may

take about three weeks to a month.

b) Abnormal cells can be passed on to one's partner.

c) Abstain from sexual intercourse after healing from a cone biopsy.

d) There may be need for a stitch around the cervix (Shirodkar suture) after one

falls pregnant to keep the cervix tightly closed and prevent miscarriage.

e)Laser treatment, Cryosurgery, Diathermy may remove the layer of

abnormal tissue

432. When is a hysterectomy considered necessary in a woman?

a) In ruptured uterus where tears are ragged and difficult to repair.
b) In severe infection of the internal female genital system.
c) To prevent spread of cancer to the uterus from adjacent organs.
d) Where there are large fibroids or numerous fibroids causing stress and discomfort in a woman whose family is complete.
e) To prevent further pregnancies

433. Which statements are true about Breast Cancer prevention?

a) Every woman from puberty onwards must have annual screening of the breasts for cancer (mammogram).

b) Mammogram is a scan of breasts to detect abnormal cells.

c) Every month a woman must examine her breasts for possible cues of abnormal growths.

d) Breast self- examination is best done after a monthly period when the breast tissue is back to normal.

e) When a woman is breast feeding, she should not be worried about unusual breast lumps or pain, or blood in breast milk.

434. Which statements are true about menopause?

a) Menopause is a stage in a woman's life when the flow of female hormones slows down gradually until it ceases.

b) Menopause is usually associated with mature women of over fifty years age group but it is known to start from the mid- forties or earlier.

c) Menopause is a gradual process except in women who have had extensive pelvic surgery.

d) Contraception can be discontinued at this time.

e) Menopause brings about changes in all the body systems.

435. Which of the following changes take place during menopause

a) The female internal genital organs reduce in size.

b) The cervix produces less mucus making the vagina less lubricated and tender.

c) Some women may experience discomfort during sexual intercourse (dyspareunia)

d) Sexual desire disappears.

e) Men's desire for sex does not decline at the same pace with women although men may be slowed down by age and ill-health.

436. There is general deterioration of amount of muscle and its texture as most women may realize that the muscle becomes flabby especially where one does not engage in exercises.

a) There may be a general feeling of fatigue.

b) The skin gradually loses its smooth texture and dries quickly requiring that

one oils the skin well frequently.

c) Hair loses its texture and colour, thins out, breaks and becomes sparse.

d) Fat is deposited around the abdomen and the hips explaining why

mature women often have large bellies.

437. How can you advise your aging mother to look after her skeletal system?

a) Bones lose their thickness and texture and become thin porous and frail making an individual prone to fractures.
b) Wear reasonable heels on shoes to prevent falls.
c) Avoid chores that require you to get onto chairs or ladders as ability to balance oneself is reduced.
d) The joints movements become reduced and you may experience stiff painful joints and may need pain relief for joint pains.
e) You can eat anything you want

438. You are training prospective carers of the elderly. Which of the statements below would be true of menopausal clients?

a) It is important that your clients eat foods that are rich in calcium and magnesium such as milk and all milk products and other minerals and vitamins from fruit and vegetables.
b) Bones thin out and become porous and fragile making your clients prone to fractures. You should limit possibilities of falls.
c) Some of your clients may feel low, irritable and moody and depressed weepy and feeling very sorry for themselves for no specific reason.
d) Expect some of your women clients to have minor to major blackouts in which they may lose orientation of time, place and people.
e) You may notice poor sleeping patterns (insomnia).

439. Which statements are true of ageing?

a) The pulse rate rises.

b) The blood vessels become rigid pipes causing the blood pressure to fall.

c) Signs of poor blood flow such as swelling of feet, breathlessness

and palpitations are likely.

d) Hearing and sight decline

e) Appetite increases and bowel movements are regular

440. Some of the treatments available for genital warts are

a) Freezing in which extremely cold rods are applied to the growth.

b) Surgical removal or by burning, cauterization

c) Antiretroviral drugs can be used to prevent recurrence of the growth.

d) Vaseline can be used for treatment

441. Sudden menopause occurs where

a) Both ovaries are removed.?

b) The uterine tubes are removed?

c) Hysterectomy or removal of the uterus is done?

d) The woman has fibroids

e) In cancer of the cervix

442. Which sexually transmitted infections present with the following:

a)   thick creamy pus
b)   thin watery pus or milky curds.
c)   Offensive watery discharge
d)   Clusters of watery discharge
e)   Crops of body rash

443. Why is it important for the midwife to examine the placenta?

a) Out of curiosity

b) To identify abnormalities in size and shape,

   membranes, blood vessels and cord insertion

c) To look for a retroplacental clot

d) To diagnose obvious abnormalities like

   infarcts suggestive of placental insufficiency

e) To report on missing lobe which could suggest retained products of pregnancy, a source of haemorrhage

444. When is it necessary to collect a specimen of cord blood?

a) When the baby looks anaemic

b) When Rh incompatibility is suspected

c) When the baby fails to cry after delivery

d) In suspected HIV mother to baby transmission

e) In delayed 2nd stage of labour.

445. What are the possible causes of urinary tract infection in the post-natal period?

a)   is associated with poor aseptic technique during labour
b)   and perineal repair,
c)   too many vaginal examinations, and
d)   inadequate treatment of urinary tract infection in pregnancy.
e)   Inadequate fluid intake

27759929R10068

Printed in Great Britain
by Amazon